The Science of Natural Healing

Mimi Guarneri, M.D., FACC

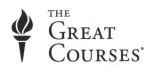

THE
GREAT
COURSES

PUBLISHED BY:

THE GREAT COURSES
Corporate Headquarters
4840 Westfields Boulevard, Suite 500
Chantilly, Virginia 20151-2299
Phone: 1-800-832-2412
Fax: 703-378-3819
www.thegreatcourses.com

Copyright © The Teaching Company, 2012

Printed in the United States of America

This book is in copyright. All rights reserved.

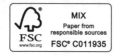

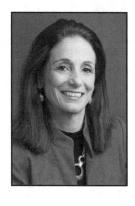

Mimi Guarneri, M.D., FACC

Founder of the Scripps Center
for Integrative Medicine

Dr. Mimi Guarneri, Founder of the Scripps Center for Integrative Medicine in California, is board certified in cardiology, internal medicine, nuclear medicine, and holistic medicine. She studied English Literature as an undergraduate at New York University, and she received her medical degree from SUNY Downstate Medical Center, where she graduated first in her class. Dr. Guarneri served her internship and residency at NewYork-Presbyterian Hospital/Weill Cornell Medical Center, where she later became Chief Medical Resident. She also completed cardiology fellowships at both NYU Langone Medical Center and Scripps Clinic.

Dr. Guarneri served as an attending physician in interventional cardiology at Scripps Clinic, where she placed thousands of coronary stents. Recognizing the need for a more comprehensive and more holistic approach to cardiovascular disease, she pioneered the Scripps Center for Integrative Medicine, where she uses state-of-the-art cardiac imaging technology and lifestyle-change programs to aggressively diagnose, prevent, and treat cardiovascular disease.

Dr. Guarneri is a member of the American College of Cardiology, the Alpha Omega Alpha Honor Medical Society, and the American Medical Women's Association. She is also a Diplomate of the American Board of Integrative Holistic Medicine and was recently elected President of the organization. In 2009, Dr. Guarneri was named Scientist of the Year by the San Diego Chapter of the Achievement Rewards for College Scientists Foundation.

Dr. Guarneri has authored several articles that have appeared in professional journals such as the *Journal of Echocardiography* and the *Annals of Internal Medicine*. She participated as a member of the writing committee for the American College of Cardiology Foundation, and in 2005, an expert consensus statement on integrating complementary medicine into cardiovascular medicine was published as a result of the committee's efforts.

Dr. Guarneri is the author of *The Heart Speaks: A Cardiologist Reveals the Secret Language of Healing*, a poignant collection of stories from cardiology patients who have benefited from integrative medicine approaches. Both *The Heart Speaks* and her clinical work have been featured on NBC's *TODAY* show and PBS's *To the Contrary* and *Full Focus*. In her book, Dr. Guarneri takes the reader on a journey of the heart—exploring the emotional heart, which capable of being crushed by loss; the intelligent heart, with a nervous system all its own; and the spiritual heart, which yearns for a higher purpose. With groundbreaking new research and unparalleled experience, Dr. Guarneri skillfully weaves the science and drama of the heart's unfolding. Her work was also featured in a two-part PBS documentary called *The New Medicine*.

Dr. Guarneri is regularly quoted in national publications such as *Yoga Journal*, *Whole Living: Body + Soul in Balance*, *Trustee* magazine and *WebMD the Magazine*. She has been recognized for her national leadership in integrative medicine by The Bravewell Collaborative and now serves as chair of the organization's Clinical Network. In 2008, she was honored by Project Concern International for her work in southern India, and she currently serves on the international subcommittee for Direct Relief International.

Dr. Guarneri also served on an advisory panel for the Institute of Medicine to explore the science and practice of integrative medicine for promoting the nation's health. The summit's findings were released in 2009 in Washington DC. ■

Table of Contents

Table of Contents

Table of Contents

Disclaimer

This course, *The Science of Natural Healing*, is intended to increase your ability to recognize medical misinformation and make use of reliable, evidence-based information when making health-related choices. These lectures are not designed for use as medical references to diagnose, treat, or prevent medical illnesses or trauma. Neither The Great Courses nor Dr. Mimi Guarneri is responsible for your use of this educational material or its consequences. If you have questions about the diagnosis, treatment, or prevention of a medical condition or illness, you should consult a qualified physician.

The Science of Natural Healing

Scope:

Western medicine focuses on disease without getting to the underlying cause, and physicians are trained to make a diagnosis and offer a drug or surgical treatment. The result is that the people of the United States are the greatest consumers of pharmaceutical therapy. It is one thing to make a diagnosis, but to offer medication without including instructions for how to reverse the disease process is shortsighted. The goal of this course is to turn this approach inside out, offering solutions to disease prevention and treatment that are embedded in how we live our lives. Treating disease after it occurs is not the solution. Once a diagnosis is made, the next obvious questions are why and how to reverse the process. Focusing on health, vitality, and longevity requires a completely different approach. Macro- and micronutrition, physical activity, herbal medicine, enhanced resiliency, and spirituality are just a few of the key components to healing. This course will explore causes of disease along with state-of-the-art biomarkers and imaging for diagnosis. Most importantly, this course will offer solutions to immediately improving many chronic problems, including arthritis and heart disease. In general, this course will offer the necessary tools to prevent disease.

This course focuses on the role of nutrition in health—offering clear guidance on eliminating common inflammation-causing and allergy-inducing foods and how to replace them with foods that lead to the production of healthy proteins. The role of herbal medicine in health, vitamins, and supplementation will be discussed, and questions regarding the right supplements, choices, and options for dosing and purity will be addressed. The course will also discuss which foods should be purchased organic and how the industrialized food system has altered nutrition options. Full programs will be offered for naturally treating diabetes, high cholesterol, and high blood pressure.

Today, many people are struggling with stress, anxiety, and depression. Acute and chronic stress affect both the physical and mental bodies of individuals; high blood pressure and high cholesterol as well as diabetes and insomnia are just a few of the effects that are experienced. One of the keys to enhancing resiliency is to change perception and practice, utilizing techniques that lead to emotional flexibility. In this course, you will explore natural approaches to stress, including breathing techniques, guided imagery, and meditation. The use of natural supplements for mental well-being along with exercise and mind-body techniques will be offered.

Throughout this course, you will explore the connection between people and the planet as you journey to an understanding of ecology and health. The choices that you make for your health are also healthy choices for the planet. From eating less dairy and meat to walking instead of driving, you will gain an understanding of how even small contributions to your health can lead to big contributions for the planet. Practical tools for improving the health of the planet while eliminating toxins, pesticides, and plastic are just a few of the topics that will be addressed.

This course will teach you everything that you need to know to stay healthy from a mind-body-spirit perspective. Whether you are seeking solutions to common diseases or wanting to achieve optimal health, this course will explore simple solutions that can be put into practice immediately. Health is our greatest wealth, and with simple tools and practical solutions, it is absolutely possible to achieve. ■

Shifting the Health-Care Paradigm
Lecture 1

As compared with the Western health-care model, the science of natural healing takes a more holistic approach to disease treatment and prevention. If you think of the human body as a tree that uses nutrients found in the soil to grow and thrive, you might be able to pinpoint maladies of the tree—the human body—by analyzing the contents of the soil—the elements that you consume and the environmental factors that surround you. This course features all of the scientific evidence and practical techniques that you will need to strengthen your soil naturally, improving your health and life.

The State of Health Care

- Physicians perform over 400,000 bypass surgeries per year and place over one million stents into clogged arteries per year. In addition, 2,200 Americans die each day of cardiovascular disease, and coronary heart disease claims one in every six deaths. Each year, approximately 795,000 people in the United States experience a new or recurrent stroke. Currently, 42.7 million women are living with some form of cardiovascular disease.

- In the United States, 2.5 trillion dollars was spent on health care last year, and it is predicted that 4.3 trillion dollars will be spent by 2023. Currently, that is 16 percent of our nation's gross domestic product, and it is double the amount of money that other developed nations spend on health care. However, despite the money that is spent, the United States is ranked 37th in the world in health outcomes.

- Much of the money that is spent on health care is spent on pharmaceutical therapy. North America consumes 47.7 percent of all the pharmaceuticals made for the entire world. In 2010, Americans spent 310 billion dollars on pharmaceutical therapy.

Acute versus Chronic Care

- Surgery and drugs are the hallmarks of Western medicine, and they definitely can be effective. Western medicine is great for acute care. For example, if you are having a heart attack or if you have just been involved in a car accident, you want to get to the best state-of-the-art Western medical facility.

- However, conventional medicine falls short in some very important areas—specifically, illness prevention and chronic disease care. Medical professionals are more trained to be reactive. In addition, they are disease driven and often only treat parts of people. For example, heart specialists are expected to just treat the heart—to treat symptoms, deal with problems as they arise, and then impose a treatment.

- There is a reason for this kind of training. Physicians are taught to ask patients one question: "What is your chief complaint?" This question already implies that the patient has a problem. Physicians then hear the chief complaint, do a physical exam, run a few tests, and quickly arrive at a diagnosis. Once they have the diagnosis, they then decide on a treatment.

- The primary training for physicians in conventional Western medicine involves arriving quickly at a diagnosis. Rapid diagnosis leads to rapid treatment, and rapid treatment can save lives. This process allows physicians to control the underlying problem.

- Problems arise when physicians take that model of acute-care medicine and apply it to chronic, long-term health issues. In addition, that model certainly does nothing to prevent illness. Instead, the clinician is taught to proceed directly to the diagnosis—to name the disease—in order to identify as quickly as possible a medication or procedure.

- When physicians apply the acute model to chronic disease, they miss a lot of information that might alert them to the cause of the problem. For example, if a patient has a headache and the physician offers a diagnosis and a prescription, the physician would be missing the essential aspects of that person's life: who they are, who they live with, what they eat, what their joys and hopes are, what their exercise regimen is, and what medications they take. Socially, the physician would not know whether they are married, belong to a community, or gain strength from their belief system.

- The result of using the acute-care model is that little attention is paid to the patient's story. Physicians are aware of the patient's chief complaint and present symptoms of illness, but the patient's whole story is not understood. Each major issue becomes a discrete diagnosis dealt with in isolation from all the others because physicians are trained to look at the parts.

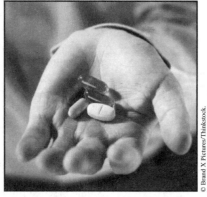

- Physicians end up with what can best be called "the ill to the pill." Everything that physicians have a diagnosis for is

Personalized medicine involves the understanding that not everyone needs the same pills for the same illnesses.

associated with a pill or a surgery because that is what is in their toolbox. The problem with this approach is that the patient ends up with a bag full of pills.

A Natural Alternative

- When it comes to the prevention and treatment of disease, nature provides the best solutions. Think of yourself as a tree that has a few health challenges. Think about the soil in which you live. You might be able to label some of the leaves of your tree—maybe as "depression," "diabetes," "high cholesterol," or "heartburn." Some people have many sick leaves.

- Imagine that the trunk of your tree is your genes—your genetic makeup. Then, think about what makes up the soil because what determines whether you have healthy or sick fruit is a very special interaction between your genes and your environment, and the soil is the environment in which you live.

- Soil ingredients interact with the trunk of your tree—with your genome—and determine if our leaves are sick or healthy. Important soil ingredients include the following.
    o Macronutrition: What kind of protein do you eat? What kind of carbohydrates do you choose? Do you eat good fats or bad fats?

    o Micronutrition: vitamins and minerals, such as vitamin D, zinc, and selenium.

    o Clean air and clean water.

    o Physical activity: Do you walk every day? Do you have a formal exercise program?

    o Sound sleep at night.

    o Environmental toxins.

- In addition to the components of the physical body, your soil has other components that are equally important: How do you live your life? How do you feel emotionally, mentally, and spiritually? Are you angry and hostile? Where is your resiliency? Do you believe in a higher power? Where do you gain your strength?

- The best way to heal your tree is by strengthening your soil. However, not everyone needs the same things. Some people need nutrition while others need exercise—and perhaps others need to reduce the amount of stress they have.

1. What is the current health-care paradigm, and how is it good for acute care?

2. Prevention and chronic disease care require a new approach to health. How do they differ from the acute-care model?

Shifting the Health-Care Paradigm
Lecture 1—Transcript

In 1994, I began my career as an interventional cardiologist. I had just finished my cardiology training in New York City, and I was really excited to be moving to sunny San Diego. Why was I excited? Because I was going to Scripps Clinic, where they were doing cutting-edge work in the treatment of coronary artery disease.

One of the procedures I was doing at Scripps was putting stents into blocked arteries. In fact, at the busiest part of my career, I was placing over 750 of these stents per year.

A stent is a metal sleeve, like the coil on a notebook. In fact, one of the first stents invented looked just like the coil on a notebook. Stents can be as small as a few millimeters. Putting a stent in an artery is a very precise technique, because usually we're not opening the whole artery, we're just opening a small section of the blood vessel. Stenting is one of the true miracles of modern medicine. It allows us to open a blockage in an artery and restore blood flow to the heart muscle in a matter of minutes. For many of my patients that meant the difference between life and death. And for many others it meant the difference between having chest discomfort with minimal activity and no chest discomfort at all.

I was fixing only small sections of a single blood vessel. But the human body is filled with blood vessels, from the bottom of our feet to the top of our head. So was I really curing heart disease? Let me give you some staggering statistics. With all these miraculous tools in our toolbox—over 400,000 bypass surgeries a year and over one million stents a year—2200 Americans die each day of cardiovascular disease. Coronary heart disease claims one in every six deaths. Each year, we have approximately 795,000 people experiencing a new or recurrent stroke. And women are not spared: 42.7 million women are currently living with some form of cardiovascular disease.

Now, another tool physicians have in their toolbox is statin therapy. Statins are cholesterol-lowering medicines that can reduce the risk of cardiovascular events. For many years, my colleagues, and even myself thought that these drugs would be a cure for heart disease. But despite all the available statin therapies on the market, large studies with thousands and thousands of patients, even if people are on statin therapy, they can still go on to have a heart attack or a stroke.

It is not that we are not spending the money. In the United States, 2.5 trillion dollars was spent on health care last year. It is predicted that $4.3 trillion will be spent by 2023. If you think about that, that is 16 percent of our nation's gross domestic product. And, it is double the amount of other developed nations. Yet, despite spending all this money, the United States ranked 37th in the world in health outcomes.

A lot of our money is being spent on pharmaceutical therapy. When we look at all the pharmaceuticals made for the entire world, North America consumes 47.7 percent. In 2010, Americans spent 310 billion dollars on pharmaceutical therapy; $13 billion was spent on statin therapy alone.

Surgery and drugs are the hallmarks of Western medicine, and they definitely can be effective. I would be the last person to tell you that Western medicine, the kind of medicine I learned in medical school, has no value. Western medicine is great for acute care. For example, if you are having a heart attack, or a stroke, or you have just had a car accident, that is when you want to get to the best state-of-the-art Western medical facility. This is what we are good at.

However, conventional medicine falls really short in some very important areas. Specifically, illness prevention and chronic disease care. We are more trained to be reactive. If you have a heart attack, we mobilize and get you taken care of. We are disease-driven. I am not even sure why we call it health care. Our focus is on disease. We treat parts of people. I am a heart specialist, so I am expected to just treat the heart. And I was trained to just treat symptoms, deal with problems when they come along, and then do a treatment.

There is a reason for this kind of training and the reason is this: As physicians, we are taught to ask of patients one question when we walk into the room, and this is a bizarre question, but it is, "What is your chief complaint? What is your problem, why are you coming here today?" It already implies you have a problem. We then hear the chief complaint, maybe do a physical exam, run a few tests, and quickly we come at a diagnosis. Once we have the diagnosis, we then decide on a treatment.

Well, this works great if your chief complaint is chest pain. You can bet you want to be in that Western medical facility if you are having a heart attack, because you are going to say "chest pain," and we are going to ask one or two other questions, quickly arrive at a diagnosis, and immediately initiate therapy, whether it is oxygen, medication, or even take you to the catheter lab for a stent. It is that quick, it is that reactive, and it is life saving.

So, our primary training in conventional Western medicine is to arrive quickly at the diagnosis. Rapid diagnosis leads to rapid treatment, and rapid treatment can save lives. It allows us to control the underlying problem; as we say, "control the physiology." So we focus on the chief complaint, we make the diagnosis, and we quickly move on.

Problems arise when we take that model of acute care medicine and we apply that to chronic, long-term health issues. And that model certainly does nothing to prevent illness. The clinician is taught to proceed directly to the diagnosis, to name the disease, in order to identify as quickly as possible a medication or a procedure.

But when we apply that model to chronic disease, look at what we are missing. If someone comes to my office and they say, "I have a headache," I make the diagnosis and I give a prescription, and I am off to my next patient. I would be missing the essential aspects of that person's life. I am missing who they are, who they live with, what they eat, what are their joys and their hopes, do they exercise, what medications do they take? There are all sorts of questions that I would be losing out on. Socially, are they married? Are they isolated? Do they have community? Do they gain strength from their belief system? All of these pieces would be missing.

The result of using the acute care model is that little attention is paid to the patient's story. What we get is the chief complaint, maybe a little bit about the present symptoms of illness. The patient's whole story is not understood. Who is this individual in context to community?

Each major issue becomes a discreet diagnosis dealt with in isolation from all the others. Remember, we were trained to look at the parts. So what do we end up with?

We end up with what can best be called, "the ill to the pill." Every ill that we have, every diagnosis that is made, we reach into our toolbox, and we take out a pill. So, for example, if someone has arthritis, we say, "Let's give you this Motrin or Aleve." If someone has high blood pressure, we give a pill for that. If someone has diabetes, we give a pill for that. If someone has heartburn—you got it—we have a pill for that. So every label that we have, everything that we have a diagnosis for, we have a pill or a surgery, because that is what is in our toolbox. The problem with the "ill to the pill" approach is you end up with a bag full of pills.

I remember the day my patient Joe came to the office. Joe was just discharged from the hospital, and he had a bag full of pills. Joe had pills for heartburn, for depression, for high blood pressure, and for diabetes. And the first thing Joe said to me was, "I do not like the way these medications make me feel. When can I get off them? Do I have any options?" Now, if Joe had come to me in the '90s when I was placing those 700 stents each year, I probably would have said, "You know what, Joe? I am afraid you really do not have options. You should be happy to be alive. You need to take your medications." Period.

But, fortunately for Joe, by the time he came to me, I actually had something of a revelation. My practice had been radically changed by a simple insight. When it comes to the prevention and treatment of disease, nature provides the best solutions.

So here is what I said to Joe. I said to Joe, "I'm not against medication, Joe." There is a time and place for medication. And I do use plenty of medicines in my patients. But I let Joe know that medication, which is great for acute care, was not necessarily the best way for him to go forward in his life. Medication was not the best way to manage each and every one of his chronic health problems. And Joe seemed really surprised. Now I had his attention, and he said to me, "You mean there really is another option?" I said, "The answer is yes. And that option is the science of natural healing." Joe looked at me and said, "What is the science of natural healing?" So to explain this concept, I drew a tree, and I asked Joe, I said, "If this was your tree and the leaves on this tree were sick, what would you do?" And without hesitation, Joe answered, he said, "I would water the tree, I would check the soil, I would make sure it was getting enough sunlight, and I even would add fertilizer. I want to strengthen the soil."

I then explained to Joe that his tree was sick, and I drew a few leaves on the tree so that Joe would be able to understand, and I labeled those leaves "diabetes," "heart disease," "heartburn," "high blood pressure." And I explained to Joe that Western medicine starts with the leaves, we go right up to the leaves, we name them, and we go for a medication or a surgery. The leaves are cut off, they are bypassed, or they are medicated. Joe seemed to understand. But, I offered Joe a different solution. "Think about this, Joe, remember what you said about the sick tree? What if we look at your soil?"

We all have a soil in which we live. And, if you take a minute, think of yourself as a tree, and you might even have a few health challenges. You might even be able to label some of the leaves of your tree, maybe one is "depression," maybe one is "diabetes," maybe a leaf on your tree is "high cholesterol," maybe it is even "heartburn." And some people have a lot of sick leaves.

Now, take your imagination a little bit further, and think about the trunk of the tree, and I want you to imagine that the trunk of that tree, of your tree, is your genes, your genetic makeup, the book of life that you were given. And now, I want you to go further. I want you to go into the soil, and I want us to look at what makes up the soil, because at the end of the day, what determines whether we have healthy or sick fruit is a very special interaction between our genes and our environment, and the soil is the environment in which we live.

Let's think about those important ingredients to the soil, the soil in which we live. They are things like macro nutrition: What kind of protein do we eat? What kind of carbohydrates do we choose? Do we eat good fats, or bad fats? What about our micronutrients, things like vitamin D, zinc, selenium? These are all part of our soil. The human body also needs clean air and clean water. Our soil is also going to be affected by our physical activity. Do we walk every day? Do we have a formal exercise program? Do we do Tai Chi? This is a key component to our soil. But it doesn't stop there. Our soil is even affected by whether or not we have sound sleep at night, and our soil is affected by environmental toxins. All of these things interact with the trunk of our tree, with our genome, and determine if our leaves are sick or healthy.

But it does not stop there. Those are just components of the physical body. Our soil has other, equally important components: How we live our lives in community, are we connected, are we socially isolated? How are we doing emotionally, mentally, spiritually? Are we angry? Are we hostile? How do we see our glass? Do we see our glass as half empty, or half full? Where is our resiliency? Do we believe in a higher power? Where do we gain our strength?

So when I think about the soil, and when I think about my soil, I have to look at all of these areas, because we know that the physical aspects of healing can't be separated from the emotional, mental, and spiritual. And all of these things which make up our soil ultimately determine whether we get sick or whether we stay well.

I spent many years stenting the branches of my patients' trees. It would not be unusual for me to wait in the cardiac catheterization lab and call over to the emergency room and say, "Is anyone there having a heart attack?" and rush in, take them to the catheterization lab, and put in a stent. In fact, it did not even faze me in the '90s when my patients would go up to the ICU and they would be eating a roast beef and mayo sandwich on white bread. In the '90s, I had a total disconnect between intervention and prevention. I never thought about it. But I have spent years learning, and I now know that we have a better way.

Whenever I talk about the ill to the pill, I think about a cartoon that I frequently use in the lectures for my patients. The cartoon is two guys in lab jackets, hospital lab coats, and they're both mopping up a mess of water that's on the floor. But there's a sink right in front of them, and the water is running from the faucet. So the water is just coming out and they're mopping up the mess. I like this cartoon because it reminds me of exactly of what I was doing. I was the one with the mop; I was mopping up the mess. I was the one that was waiting for someone to come with a heart attack, and then I would go in and put in a stent. It never occurred to me at the time that what I really needed to be doing was reaching up and turning off the faucet.

I now know that the best way to heal the tree, to heal your tree, is by strengthening your soil. Not everyone needs the same thing. For some, it is nutrition, for others it is exercise, and maybe for someone else it is stress reduction. And some of us need a few of these things.

In this course I will share with you all of the scientific evidence and practical techniques that you will need to strengthen your own soil.

Understanding Holistic Integrative Medicine
Lecture 2

olistic integrative medicine is a new paradigm for health care that completely reverses the old paradigm; it's a whole new philosophy. Traditional Western physicians are trained to believe that the foundation of health care involves drugs and surgery. On the other hand, holistic integrative practitioners are trained to take care of the whole person—body, mind, and spirit—and to understand a patient's connection to his or her community. Holistic integrative medicine is about food, love, touch, micro- and macronutrition, moving and exercise, and prayer and meditation.

What Is Holistic Integrative Medicine?
- Using the holistic integrative medicine model of care, physicians do not just treat symptoms—they get to the underlying cause. They do not just treat the physical body; they do not separate the emotional, mental, and spiritual aspects of healing from the physical.

- In essence, holistic integrative physicians create a bridge between the best of global healing traditions. For example, they combine yoga, meditation, and vegetarian diet, which are components of Ayurvedic medicine from India. However, patients still take their medications—they engage in both concepts together. As a result, a bridge is created between Ayurvedic medicine and Western medicine.

- Integrative holistic medicine is not about alternative medicine, which implies taking an alternative route to mainstream medicine. In alternative medicine, a patient might choose to do diet and nutrition-infusion therapies and not to do chemotherapy and radiation.

- With integrative holistic medicine, physicians use a combination of all of the treatment options available. If you need a bypass, chemo, or radiation, then you will be subjected to those methods, but these physicians will also do the best that they can to add methods used in global healing traditions, including yoga and meditation.

- The term "holistic" just means "whole," and in this context, it involves treating the whole person—not just a small part. It means looking at the physical but also looking at the mental, emotional and spiritual. It is embracing the individual in the world and environment in which they live, including the people that surround them and their connection to the planet.

- If you have a chair that has four legs on it, the chair needs those four legs to be balanced—or it will tip over. Think about the four legs as body, mind, emotion, and spirit. Each of us needs to do something in every category every day to remain balanced. Some people need a little more in one place than another, but it is all needed for wholeness, health, and healing.

- Global healing traditions are traditions that have been around for many thousands of years. An example is traditional Chinese medicine, which has been around for over 5,000 years. It has a philosophy and an education: To become a doctor of Chinese medicine, you must complete as rigorous a training program as any medical school training program.

- Another global healing tradition is Ayurvedic medicine, which comes from India and is also over 5,000 years old. You become an Ayurvedic physician when you train in India in that discipline. It focuses on nutrition and on keeping people well using massage and oils, yoga, and meditation.

- In the world of holistic integrative medicine, doctors are teachers who teach about prevention, health, and wellness. It is about being a healer. It is about being present with patients and partnering with patients. Healing a patient's life requires getting to the underlying issues and working them through.

- Happiness, which many physicians are not even taught about in medical school, can no longer be ignored. In addition, death is part of the human process. That does not mean that physicians should not do everything they can to keep you healthy and well, but they should not view death as a failure.

- Emotional and physical pain—and even mental and spiritual pain—are not the enemies. Sometimes, pain is a teacher; sometimes, it is a lesson. Sometimes, it is a warning that something is out of balance.

Principles of Integrative Holistic Medicine

- Integrative holistic medicine physicians and practitioners believe that prevention is the best intervention. Prevention, getting to the underlying cause of disease, is what distinguishes this model from traditional Western medicine.

- When using holistic integrative medicine, physicians focus on optimal health, which is the conscious pursuit of the highest level of

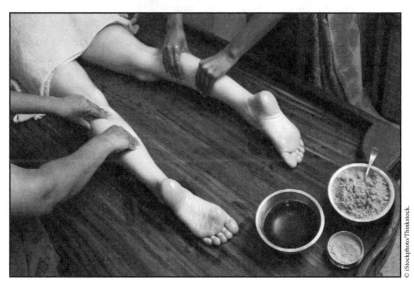

Ayurvedic medicine, which stems from India, involves the use of massage and oils to keep people well.

functioning that can be obtained—a balance between the physical, mental, emotional, spiritual, and environmental and social aspects of being human.

- It does not matter where you begin; everyone is in a different spot on the journey to optimal health. In addition, one size does not fit all; not everyone needs the same meditation program, yoga program, or pill. Physicians need to look at people as individuals and engage in personalized medicine, which focuses on the unique aspects of an individual—on the nature of the person.

- Holistic medicine physicians partner with their patients, get to the underlying cause, recognize the individuality of each patient, and embrace the wisdom found in all the global healing traditions.

- One of the deep core principles of integrative holistic medicine is about the fundamentals of life. Physicians recognize that all experiences in life, birth, joy, suffering, and even dying are profound opportunities for learning.

- Physicians who use the integrative holistic medicine model also know that they have an innate power to heal. In fact, all people have the ability to heal; we just have to tap into the wisdom of the body, the body's innate power, and bring that forth. We cannot tap into that—to fight an infection or cancer, for example—if we are stressed out because stress suppresses our immune system. One of the goals of integrative holistic physicians is to help people utilize these powers to put them into the right space for healing.

- Finally, love is the most powerful healer. One of the most important things that physicians can do for their patients, in partnership with their patients, is to meet each individual with kindness, acceptance, and grace—not judgment.

1. What is the philosophy of holistic integrative medicine?

2. How does holistic integrative medicine differ from conventional Western medical care?

Understanding Holistic Integrative Medicine
Lecture 2—Transcript

In 1996, I was having a typical day in the cardiac catheterization lab. I was placing stents, doing angioplasty, and I will never forget this: I opened the door to the lab, walked out, and standing there was a guy named Dean Ornish. Now, I did not know who Dr. Ornish was. I did not know about his research, did not know about the books that he wrote. I did not know anything about him. And he said to me, "I have been told that you would be perfect to do some research in heart patients." And I said, "Great!" I really thought that he was going to say, "I have a new stent," or "I have a new angioplasty catheter," but instead what he said to me was, "I want to take some of your sickest heart patients, people that are not even candidates for bypass or stenting"—now these are really sick people. And he said, "I want you to teach them yoga. I want you to teach them meditation, exercise, place them on a vegetarian diet, and put them in support groups." "Well I have to be honest," I said to Dr. Ornish, "With all due respect,"—those were my exact words—"I don't know anything about yoga, I know less about meditation, I surely do not know anything about vegetarian diet, and I definitely am not a psychologist and I can't run a support group. I was not taught this in medical school, I was taught to do what I am doing now." To his credit, he just laughed. He said, "You know what? I was trained in the same way you were. But I still want you to do the research."

So I decided that if I was going to do a research study that involved yoga and meditation, I needed to know something about this. I mean, how could I be a principle investigator on a research study and not know anything about what I was studying?

So I decided to participate in the study basically as a patient. I took my own cholesterol level, drew my own blood, went to the yoga classes, and started to do everything that the patients did. If you can imagine, we took these really sick heart patients who were told by surgeons, "You can't have a bypass, you will never make it." And then in the '90s, we did not have the kind of stents we have today, today I call stents "heat seeking missiles," they can go right into the blood vessel. We used to struggle for hours in the '90s to get a stent in.

I began on this path to do the research side-by-side with my patients. They came in three times a week, sometimes for as much as four hours a day, and together we did yoga, we learned to meditate, the patients sat in support groups, talked about their stories. This went on for over a year. The results were amazing. In fact, they were astonishing. The obvious things occurred: People lost weight—that is true; their diabetes got better; they were able to get rid of a lot of their medications. But something even more important than that happened. What was really fascinating to me was that people transformed their lives. I never thought of heart disease as a family disease. When someone is really sick—it does not have to be heart disease—with any disease, the whole family is involved. I heard spouses talk to me about walking on eggshells, afraid if they did something their partner, their husband, or their wife, would have a heart attack. The transformation I saw was not only in the patients, it was in the kids, it was in the spouses, it was in the entire family.

When we concluded the research we saw people were less depressed, they responded differently to stressful situations, their relationships got better, even more importantly they started to ask really deep questions like, "What is my purpose in life?" And, "If I do have something that is physically wrong, how do I want to spend the next time on this planet?" "Do I want to be arguing with my neighbor?" Or, "Do I want to be with my grandkids?" The list was endless, and as a physician, I was completely transformed.

I have never, and will never, be the same cardiologist. There is no way after what I witnessed—the changes in people's lives through this research, the healing on a mind, body, and spirit level that was accomplished—there is no way that I can go back to just saying I can cure coronary disease with a stent and a drug. I knew beyond a shadow of a doubt that that was simply not true. I knew with all my heart that I needed to take up the mission and to create a new model of health care. And the model that I embraced was what we call, today, Holistic Integrative Medicine.

In this model of care, we do not just treat symptoms; we get to the underlying cause. We do not just treat the physical body; we do not separate the emotional, mental, and spiritual aspects of healing from the physical.

What we did, in essence, was we created a bridge. It was a bridge between the best of global healing traditions. For example, for the Ornish research, we used yoga and meditation and vegetarian diet. That comes right out of Ayurvedic medicine from India. But our patients still got their medications, we did not stop their drugs, we did not stop their aspirin and things that they needed for their heart, we did both together. A bridge was created between Ayurvedic medicine and Western medicine. Integrative medicine is all about that bridge: How can we use the best from both worlds to bring about healing?

For me, personally, I became a bridge physician. I began to feel as comfortable talking about vegetarian diet because—guess what?—I myself became a vegetarian. I can't teach vegetarian diet if I am not a vegetarian; that does not make sense. So I can feel as comfortable teaching vegetarian diet as I feel recommending a bypass. Or as comfortable recommending omega-3 fish oil and meditation as I feel recommending some tried and true heart medicines like Coreg or kinase inhibitors. I will go back and forth between both worlds, not only in my practice but also with my colleagues. I can stand in front of a conference filled with heart specialists and talk exactly about these things because I have developed a new language that lives in both worlds.

Integrative Holistic Medicine is not about alternative medicine. Alternative medicine implies I am going to do an alternative to mainstream medicine. In alternative medicine, I would see a patient choose to do diet and nutrition infusion therapies and maybe not do their chemotherapy and radiation. But, in Integrative Holistic Medicine, we use it all. If you need a bypass, if you need chemo, if you need radiation, we do all of those things. But we also do the best that we can with picking from the global healing traditions, whether it is yoga, or meditation, and so on.

I feel it is important to go through some of the terms and concepts, because even my own colleagues do not know what they mean. I remember years ago being at a conference, and I used the word "holistic," and I saw some eyebrows going up because some of my colleagues equate holistic medicine with snake oil, or that I am going to be doing something really unusual, and I just tell them, Guess what, guys? Holistic just means whole—treating the whole person, not just one little part. I am not a parts person. It means looking at the physical, but also looking at the mental, emotional, and spiritual. It is embracing the individual in the world in which they live and the environment that they live in, the people that surround them and their connection to the planet. That is what holistic means.

I like to teach it to my patient this way. I tell my patients if you have a chair, and the chair has four legs on it, you need those four legs to be balanced or the chair will tip over, everybody knows that. So I like them to think about the four legs as body, mind, emotions, and spirit. And a day doesn't go by where I don't ask my patients, "What did you do for body, mind, emotions, and spirit today?" Because each of us needs to do something in every category. Some of us need a little more in one place than another, but it is all needed for wholeness, for health, and for healing.

Let's take a look at what we mean by integrative medicine. I mentioned the term earlier: global healing traditions. What does that mean? Global healing traditions are traditions that have been around, many for thousands of years. An example would be traditional Chinese medicine. Traditional Chinese medicine has been around for over 5000 years. It has a philosophy, it has an education, you become a doctor of Chinese medicine, it is as rigorous a training as any medical school training that I have gone through. Another global healing tradition would be Ayurvedic medicine, which comes from India. Again, over 5000 years old. And you become an Ayurvedic physician when you train in India in that discipline. And it focuses on things like nutrition, on keeping people well using massage and oils, yoga and meditation, lots of pieces that we used, for example, in our clinical trial.

So integrative medicine says I will keep the global healing tradition of Western medicine, because that is a global healing tradition, and I will enhance it. I will bring in all these other pieces, whatever it takes to get my patient well.

I did not name all of the global healing traditions, and I certainly do not mean to leave anyone out, because we have only homeopathy, naturopathy, there are many, including Western medicine, and many physicians today are now trained in one or the other. I know many physicians who are trained, for example, in Ayurvedic medicine, or who are trained in traditional Chinese medicine, and they, too, are bridge people.

Let's think a little bit about the concept of holistic and integrative together. Because you can put acupuncture needles in someone and say you are an acupuncturist, and do integrative medicine, but do you know something about that person? Are you taking care of them body, mind, and spirit? Is your approach holistic? That is no different than my giving Lipitor, or a drug, and not getting to the underlying cause of a problem. So when I say "holistic integrative medicine," what I am talking about is a whole new philosophy.

In the first lecture, I really talked about being trained as a repairman. As a physician, I was taught: Go to the emergency room, get the patient having the heart attack, put in the stent. But as a holistic integrative medicine physician, I am thrilled that my role has changed. The word doctor, for example, means teacher. To teach and to teach about prevention, about health, about wellness, this is one of my missions. It is about being a healer. It is about being present with my patients, and partnering with my patients. The days are over where I tell a patient do as I say, not as I do. I need to be a model of health. I need to meet my patients where they are at. I can't focus any more on just fixing broken parts, as a holistic integrative physician, I am looking at the whole person. Healing one's life requires getting to the underlying issues and working them through.

I used to think that my job was done if I gave a pill and I got an expected result. I used to think that if someone had high blood pressure, and I gave them medicine and the blood pressure came down, I got the result, I am happy, the patient is happy. I was not really focusing on anything else. I was not really looking at what mattered in that patient's life.

Do you know, very few people come to me and say, "My primary objective is to get my LDL down." They may say, "I would like to lower my cholesterol," but ultimately they say, "I want to feel better. I want to be happier. I want to spend time with my grandkids. I want to see my nephew graduate from high school. I want to be at my daughter's wedding." This is what I hear in my practice. So happiness, which I was never even taught about in medical school, can no longer be ignored.

I also was taught that if a patient died, that we failed; that as physicians, we did not do our job. And we always felt bad about it. I remember once when I was an intern at Cornell, and I had a lady in the ICU for six months, and I worked on this woman every day. I wasn't partnering with her; she was in the ICU on a ventilator. Every day, I would go in and put IVs in and order medications, and one day she opened her eyes, and she said, "I want to die." "Oh my God," I thought, "I can't handle this. I wasn't trained to handle this. My training is for you to live." And I have come to realize that death is part of the human process. That doesn't mean we don't do everything to keep you healthy and well, but I no longer see it as a failure.

And one of the biggest lessons I learned practicing Integrative Holistic Medicine is that the concept of pain, emotional pain, physical pain, even mental and spiritual pain, they are not the enemies. You know, we're trained that if someone has pain, we give a painkiller. We do not ask the question, "Why is someone in pain? What is that about?" Sometimes pain is a teacher. Sometimes it is a lesson. Sometimes it is a warning; it is telling us something is out of balance, pay attention. This is the way we think as integrative holistic physicians.

Let's take a look at some of the big principles, and the same principles I am going to share with you today I share with physicians. I teach this exact lecture, or close to it, to physicians every year who are dissatisfied with their practice and want to do something different.

What does it mean to be an Integrative Holistic Medicine physician and practitioner? Well one of the first things we believe in is that prevention is the best intervention. You have heard me say in a previous lecture, when you need a stent in the acute emergency of a heart attack, we absolutely want to have that technology available to us. I do not want to throw the baby out with the bathwater. I want to have the technology available. But prevention, getting to the underlying cause of disease, this is what distinguishes us from traditional Western medicine. We don't just say, "You have diabetes, here is your pill," we say, "You have diabetes, and let's explore why."

I like to share one little story. I had a patient come to see me with high blood pressure, and he said to me he had been to four different physicians, and every physician gave him a different blood pressure pill. And he went through all the tests to find out if he had something unusual about him that led to that high blood pressure. And all those tests came back normal, any yet, every time he got a new medicine. So now he is on four blood pressure pills—that is a lot. So I said, "Well, Let's take a look at what is going on." I said, "Let's just look through your day, first. Let's start in the morning. I want you to tell me everything you do, from when you get up to when you go to bed." I said to this patient, "I want you to tell me what you eat, who you eat with, what you drink, how you prepare your food, I want to go through everything." And the answer came right away. This man was drinking 15 bottles of electrolyte water a day. Now I will not name names, but he was drinking electrolytes filled with—what?—sodium. Fifteen bottles a day. "Oh," I said, "your blood pressure is easy to fix, give up that drink. Come and see me next week." Needless to say, his blood pressure was cured. If I didn't ask him what he was eating, I would not have gotten to the underlying cause of his high blood pressure.

Let's take a look at another principle. We do not really focus on quantity of life in holistic integrative medicine; we really focus on optimal health. Optimal health is one of our primary goals. What does optimal health mean? It is the conscious pursuit of the highest level of functioning we can obtain. It does not matter where we start. Everyone is in a different place. Everyone is in a different spot on the journey. But it is the highest level of functioning and a balance between the physical, the mental, the emotional, the spiritual, and also the environmental and social aspects of being human. This is what it means to be optimally healthy. When I think about it, if I am at my peak, and I am healthy, I am going to have happiness. It is about social connection, about our family, community, and for many of us, a connection to a higher power, whether that is nature, the divine, or some other belief system. Emotionally, we feel confident, we feel good about who we are. Physically, we have good energy, our vitality is up, we are in harmony with our surroundings, and probably one of the most important pieces is we have peace of mind, because as you will hear in later lectures, if we have peace of mind, we are less likely to go and look for peace in unhealthy foods, in cigarettes, in drugs, and other things like that. This is what it means to be optimally healthy.

We all know that not one size fits all, not everyone needs the same thing. Not everyone needs the same meditation program, or yoga program, not everyone needs the same pill. We need to look at people as individuals. We call it personalized medicine. We focus on the unique aspects of an individual, on the nature of the person. A great and brilliant physician, Sir William Osler said this: "It is much more important to know what type of person has the disease than what disease a person has." I will say that again, because it is so key: "It is more important to know what type of person has a disease not just what disease a person has."

What else do we do? What else makes us different? We partner with our patients, we get to the underlying cause, we recognize the individuality of each and every one of us, and we embrace the wisdom found in all the global healing traditions. I talked a bit about this earlier. It is no longer just one or two tools in my toolbox. Now I have a toolbox filled with tools, so when that patient comes in and is depressed, I do not tell them, "Here is your antidepressant," that is not my first reaction. I am going to say, "Let's get to the underlying cause of that depression. Let's get to the underlying cause of your arthritis." I can tell you right now, and we will talk about this in later lectures, if you have arthritis, there is a good chance you are eating the wrong foods. Let's take a look at that. So now I can go into my toolbox, and say, "Let's get you on the right herbal remedies that prevent inflammation. Let's get you on the right foods that prevent inflammation. Let's get you some massage and some acupuncture." Now my toolbox is filled with tools, which, by the way, are evidence-based. This is not just pie-in-the-sky medicine. They are evidence-based tools, embedded in science, in the right situation to help people heal.

Now, one of the deep core principles of Integrative Holistic Medicine is about the fundamentals of life. We recognize that all experiences in life, birth, joy, suffering, even dying, are profound opportunities for learning. As I said before, being with my patient in that ICU, I learned a lot about dying. She taught me a lot about dying. I did not learn it in medical school.

We also know that we have within ourselves the innate power to heal. All people have the ability to heal; we just have to tap into the wisdom of the body, the body's innate power, and to bring that forth. We can't tap into that if we are stressed out, stress suppresses our immune system, we can't fight infection, we can't fight cancer. So one of our goals as integrative holistic physicians is to help people utilize these powers, to tap into them, to put them into the right space for healing. If we cut our hand, do we have to tell our hand, "Oh, heal up, bring in the white cells, bring in the fibroblasts." No, the body already knows how to do it; we just need to access the knowing.

Finally, we believe that love is the most powerful healer. I will tell you, if I thought 15 years ago that I would be giving this lecture saying that love is the most powerful healer, I would have laughed. And yet, I see it every day in my practice that one of the most important things I can do for my patients, with my patients, in partnership with my patients, is to open my heart and to come from love—not to come from judgment—to meet each individual with kindness, with acceptance, with grace.

One of my heroes is Mother Theresa. And Mother Theresa had this to say: "It is not how much you do, but how much love you put into the doing that matters."

We could fill our day up with lots of things to do, but remember to put some love into it, no matter how small we think it is. It is not how much you do, but how much you do with intention and from the heart.

So we have a new paradigm for health care, and the new paradigm turns the old paradigm upside-down. I was trained to have the foundation of health care be drugs and surgery. If you think about a pyramid, the bottom, the base of the pyramid, was specialists and drugs and operations. Now, that is the top of the pyramid, the apex. The base of the pyramid is about taking care of the whole person, about body, mind, and spirit, about connection, connection to community. It's about food, it's about love, it's about touch, it's about micro and macro nutrition, it's about moving and exercise, it's about prayer and meditation. We have completely shifted the thinking and Integrative Holistic Medicine has made this, for me as a physician, completely possible.

You Are More Than Your Genes
Lecture 3

In this lecture, you will learn about some of the fascinating research that has been done on the human genome, and you will explore the new fields of nutrigenomics and pharmacogenomics. Even more importantly, you will learn that it is possible to turn genes on and off through nutrition and lifestyle change. Nutrients and the environment in which you live can influence your epigenome and, ultimately, your health. Throughout the rest of this course, you will be given the tools to make nutrition and lifestyle choices that can have positive and profound impacts on your genes.

Genes Plus Environment

- The first survey of the entire human genome, called the Human Genome Project, determined that the genome had far fewer genes than were anticipated, but the variation of the genes was far greater than expected—with over three million variations.

- Our phenotype—how we look—results from an interaction of our genes and our environment. This interaction occurs through what is called the epigenome.

- Human beings have 23 chromosomes, and they occur in pairs. One member of each pair comes from your father, and one comes from your mother.

- Our epigenome is a personal history of our life from conception to death, and the composition of this epigenome is the result of our genetic determinants—our lineage—and our environment.

- According to Randy Jirtle, an authority on the epigenome, certain genes appear more epigenetically sensitive than others, and it is clear in the fetus that these genes are capable of being environmentally marked.

- Researchers use a mouse called the Agouti mouse—which is yellow, fat, and has a high risk of cancer, diabetes, and obesity—to study these diseases. If a pregnant Agouti mouse is given nutrients such as zinc and the B vitamins known as folate and B12, the mom produces a completely normal offspring. The baby is thin, brown, and has no risk, or a much lower risk, of cancer, diabetes, and obesity, and the baby mouse lives a long life.

- This has profound implications: What we do not only affects our own epigenome, but it also affects the next generation. When a mom eats during pregnancy, she is imprinting the fetus with information—called epigenetic tags. There are many conditions that are associated with these tags, including type 2 diabetes, heart disease, autoimmune disease, Alzheimer's disease, allergies, and even some cancers.

- All of these major medical conditions can be influenced by environmental factors. Our chances of developing any or all of these conditions can be increased or decreased by how we live our lives. In other words, your genes are not your destiny; you are more than your genes.

- A number of vitamins, minerals, and phytochemicals—which are chemicals that come from plants—have been shown to affect the epigenome. For example, niacin, zinc, iron, riboflavin, and resveratrol can affect the epigenome.

- We take in nutrients all day. The food that we eat is metabolized, and it is absorbed by our small intestine. Eventually, it is broken down, goes into our bloodstream, and enters the cells of our body. The nutrients, which are the breakdown products of whatever we ate, sit on top of the epigenome and tell the epigenome to turn specific genes on or off, expressing different kinds of proteins.

Genetic-Environmental Research

- When genetically identical twins grow up, they do not always have the same diseases. One may have cancer, for example, and the other may not.

- In 2008 in the *Archives of Internal Medicine*, a study was published that looked at a gene called the FTO obesity gene. Researchers studied a population that has this genetic variant to be obese: the Amish people. However, when they evaluated the community, they were not obese. The members of the Amish community were walking over 18,000 steps per day, so the obesity gene was trumped by physical activity.

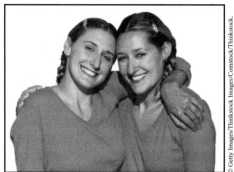

Even though genetically identical twins may appear to be the same person, they do not always contract the same diseases.

- Numerous studies have shown that there are incredibly strong links between chronic stress and poor health. Stress is a recognized risk factor for a number of diseases, including diabetes, heart disease, and high blood pressure.

- Telomeres are DNA proteins that are essential to cell division. Our cells are dividing all the time, and we change our full body every seven years or so; we do not have the same cells we were born with. Without telomeres, we would not be able to make new cells, so we would die. Telomerase is the enzyme involved in this crucial mechanism.

- In one study, Dr. Elizabeth Blackburn evaluated the relationship between stress and aging on telomeres and telomerase to determine if stress impacts health by affecting the rate of cellular aging. She

31

measured the telomere length and the telomerase enzyme in 58 premenopausal women and found that women who had the highest levels of perceived stress had the shortest telomeres. In essence, these high-stress women had a cell age that was 10 years older than their biological age.

Nutrigenomics and Pharmacogenomics

- An emerging field called nutrigenomics involves the study of the relationship between genes and nutrition.

- The ApoE is a type of genotype that is tested routinely in heart patients. We inherit one of these genes from each of our parents. The ApoE has three different types: ApoE2, ApoE3, and ApoE4. Most of us are born with the E3 variant. The E4 variant predicts the highest risk for heart disease and Alzheimer's disease. Those individuals with the E2 variant do better on a high-fat diet, but those with the E4 variant do better on a low-fat diet.

- There is not one diet that fits all because everyone is unique. However, we now have genetic information that is going to start to tell us what kind of nutrition recommendations that we should make.

- Nutritionists are being trained in this area because they are getting ready for what is called the nutrigenomics revolution, which would involve physicians making recommendations about what a person should eat and which supplements or drugs to take based on his or her specific genes.

- Another area of amazing promise is pharmacogenomics, which involves the study of the interaction between medication and genes. Physicians are already starting to put this information into clinical practice.

- Statins are drugs that lower cholesterol, and there is a genetic blood test that can tell you whether you are prone to have a problem with metabolism of statins. When certain people in the population take a statin cholesterol-lowering drug, they get muscle aches, joint aches, and pain. If you are at risk for this problem, then you should try other medications that are not statin therapy.

Questions to Consider

1. What is the epigenome?

2. What are some potential lifestyle changes that can affect the epigenome?

You Are More Than Your Genes
Lecture 3—Transcript

June 26, 2000 is a historic day in American history because on this day President Clinton stood side-by-side with J. Craig Venter and Francis Collins to announce the completion of the first survey of the entire human genome.

What we learned from the Human Genome Project was this: The genome actually had far fewer genes than were anticipated, but the variation of the genes was far greater than anyone expected, with over three million variations. Our phenotype, what we express, how we look, for example, results from an interaction of our genes and our environment. This interaction occurs through what is called the epigenome.

I like to think about it this way: We all have 23 chromosomes. They are in pairs. One member of each pair comes from dad, and one comes from mom. I like to think of this as our 23 chapters in our book of life, because what we express and who we are depends on what chapter we read.

Let me explain this. If my arm is DNA, my genetic material, the sleeve that washes over my arm is the epigenome. Epi- means above. Basically what I am saying is the epigenome washes over the genes, and the epigenome is influenced by how we live our lives, the food we eat, the stress levels that we have, the nutrients that we take.

Let me give you another visual. If the gene is my arm, and the epigenome is what washes over my genes, I like to think about drops of rain falling down on the epigenome, but those drops of rain are really information, and that information is coming from things like our nutrients, which then go and influence the epigenome resulting in certain genes being turned on and certain genes being turned off.

What this means is that our epigenome is really a personal history of our life from conception to death, and the composition of this epigenome is a result of our genetic determinants, our lineage, and as we just said, our environment.

According to Randy Jirtle, an authority on the epigenome, certain genes appear more, what is described as epigenetically sensitive, than others.

It is clear in the fetus that these genes are capable of being environmentally marked. Let me give you another example. Researchers have a mouse called the Agouti mouse. The Agouti mouse is yellow, it's fat, and it has a high risk of cancer, diabetes, and obesity. It has a reduction in its lifespan. So this mouse is used in research to study these diseases. If we take a pregnant Agouti mouse and we give the mom nutrients like zinc, and the B vitamins, folate and B12, the mom produces a completely normal offspring. The baby is thin, is brown, and has no risk, or a much lower risk, of cancer, diabetes, and obesity, and the baby mouse lives a long life. This has profound implications. Let's just stop and think about this for a second. A pregnant mouse is being given nutrients and the nutrients that mom eats affects the baby mouse developing cancer, diabetes, and obesity. What we are saying here is not only what we do affects our own epigenome, but what we do also affects the next generation.

The nutrient signature imprints us with information. What that is saying is that when a mom eats during pregnancy she is imprinting the fetus with information, which are now called epigenetic tags. We now know that there are many conditions that are associated with these epigenetic tags. These include things that we see every day in health-care, like type II diabetes, heart disease. We also see these epigenetic tags involved in autoimmune disease, in Alzheimer's disease, allergies, and even in some cancers.

All of these major medical conditions can be influenced by environmental factors. Our chances of developing any or all of these conditions can be increased or decreased by how we live our lives. In other words what I am saying is your genes are not your destiny. You are more than your genes.

We already know that a number of vitamins and minerals and phytochemicals, which are chemicals that come from plants, have been shown to affect the epigenome. We saw in the baby mouse that when the baby received the B vitamins, the mouse came out normal. What else do we know about these vitamins and nutrients? Things like niacin, zinc, iron, riboflavin, even resveratrol, which comes in dark red grapes, can affect the epigenome. So what this translates into is food is really information.

The *Journal of Clinical Nutrition* reported that diet induced changes in the epigenome during pregnancy and early development may increase the risk of the metabolic syndrome which is a condition associated with diabetes.

Imagine, diet-induced changes during pregnancy or early development can predict risk of a disease maybe 20 or 35 years later. And, as we said, even can predict risk in the next generation.

This is so important that I just want to review one piece again. We take in nutrients all day long. The food that we eat is metabolized, and it is absorbed by our small intestine. Eventually it gets into our bloodstream; it is broken down, and goes into our bloodstream and enters the cells of our body. Our cells are not seeing a ham sandwich, but our cells are seeing the breakdown products of whatever we ate. Our cells are seeing things like folate, for example, if we ate lots of green leafy vegetables. These nutrients, like those drops of rain, sit on top of the epigenome and tell the epigenome, "Turn this gene on, or that gene off." When we turn a gene on, or a gene off, we express different kinds of proteins.

Now let's take a look at the research that highlights this interaction between our genes and our environment. The most obvious one to talk about is twins, genetically identical twins. When we see them, we can't even separate them apart. Usually only mom or dad knows which one is which. But we know that when the twins grow up, they don't always have the same diseases in mid life. One may have cancer, for example, and the other may not. I have a dear friend who is a genetically identical twin, and her sister had a heart attack at the age of 36. This sent my friend into an uproar, because she thought she was next. But I explained to her, I said, "Your sister was smoking three packs of cigarettes every day. You need to do everything you can do to place your genes in a different environment, because research is showing us that the epigenome is involved."

In the *Archives of Internal Medicine* in 2008, a study was published that looked at a gene called the FTO obesity gene. They studied a population that has this genetic variant to be obese. They studied the Amish people. But when they evaluated the community, they were not obese. And what they concluded was that the members of the Amish community were walking over 18,000 steps a day. The obesity gene in this case was trumped by physical activity.

That is pretty profound, because if something like physical activity could almost silence a gene that is predisposing us to something like diabetes or obesity, then that exercise becomes very powerful medicine.

Let me share another study with you. Dr. Dean Ornish has done a lot of research in heart disease. But he decided to apply similar principles to men with low-grade prostate cancer. What he did was he taught men how to eat a very low-fat, plant-based, whole foods diet, so he changed their entire diet. He put them in stress management classes where they learned yoga and meditation. He got them exercising, and he put them in social support groups to help deal with stress. He did this for just three months. The men were biopsied before, and they were biopsied again after the three-month lifestyle intervention. And what they found was amazing: Biopsies after the intervention showed that over 400 genes associated with prostate cancer were turned off. This is only a three-month intervention, to turn off prostate cancer genes. Again, this is very powerful medicine.

Some of the most fascinating studies are coming out in the arena of stress. Numerous studies have shown that there are incredibly strong links between chronic stress and poor health. Stress is a recognized risk factor for a number of diseases: diabetes, heart disease, high blood pressure—and the list goes on.

Telomeres are DNA proteins that are essential to cell division. Our cells are dividing all the time. We change our full body every seven years or so. We do not have the same cells we were born with. Without telomeres, we would not be able to make new cells, and obviously, we would die. Telomerase is the enzyme involved in this crucial mechanism.

In a study conducted by Dr. Elizabeth Blackburn, she evaluated the relationship between stress and aging on telomeres and telomerase. I want to mention that Dr. Blackburn received the Nobel Prize for her work. In this one study, she took 58 pre-menopausal women and she had them fill out questionnaires about stress in their life, how they see the world, how they perceive themselves as stressed. Dr. Blackburn wanted to determine if stress impacts health by affecting the rate of cellular aging. She then went ahead and measured the telomere length and the telomerase enzyme.

I like to think about it this way: Imagine you have a shoelace, and at the end of the shoelace is a plastic tip. That plastic tip is your telomere, and over time, the tip could wear down and it can break down. Well as the telomere tip breaks down, so do we age, and the more broken down it is, the closer we are to death.

Now what did she find? Those women who had the highest levels of perceived stress have the shortest telomeres. In essence, these high-stress women had a cell age that was 10 years older than their biological age. It was 10 years older than the cell age of the low-stress women. Now have we not all seen this? Have we not said, "Boy, that person has really aged under stress?" This incredible finding for the first time begins to unlock the secret to stress and aging.

How else might we use this genetic information for practical purposes? The most profound thing that we talked about up until this point is that nutrients and food and the environment in which we live, can influence the epigenome and ultimately our health. And that, in and of itself, is an amazing story.

But a new field is emerging, called nutrigenomics. Just like the name sounds, nutrigenomics is studying the relationship between genes and nutrition; genes and the food that we eat. Let me give you an example that we use already in cardiology today. The ApoE is a type of genotype which is tested routinely in heart patients. We inherit one of these genes from each of our parents. The ApoE has three different types: ApoE2, ApoE3, and ApoE4. Let me stop there for a second. The ApoE3 is the one we see in the majority of people. The ApoE4 predicts the highest risk for heart disease and Alzheimer's disease. And I want us to remember, if you go out and have this blood test tomorrow, if you are an ApoE4, please do not run around and say, "I'm going to get heart disease or Alzheimer's disease." This is just a predictor of risk; this is not a diagnosis.

So how does knowing something about the ApoE4, 3, and 2 relate at all to nutrition? Well, most of us are born, as I said, with the E3 variant. However, those individuals with the E2 variant actually do better on a high-fat diet, especially if they have a problem in their blood called high triglycerides, which is a form of fat. Now, individuals with the E4 variant do better with a really low-fat diet, 20 percent versus 35 percent.

As a cardiologist, I have known for years that there is not one diet that fits all. Everyone is unique and different. But imagine that we now have genetic information that is going to start to tell us what kind of nutrition recommendations that we should make.

Nutritionists already, in this country, are being trained in this area, because they are getting ready for what is called the nutrigenomics revolution, which is when we can really start saying to people, based on X, Y, and Z genes, this is how you should eat, these are the supplements you should take, and as you will see in a minute, the drugs you should take or avoid.

Which brings us to another area of amazing promise, and that is pharmacogenomics. And as this name implies, this field studies the interaction between medication and genes. We are already starting to put this information into clinical practice. Let's take a look at how.

There is a drug that we commonly use in cardiology called warfarin. Its other name is Coumadin. Coumadin is a blood thinner, and it is metabolized by liver enzymes. When I have to put a patient on Coumadin, I never quite know what dose to give, because everyone metabolizes this drug differently. And that is kind of scary, because as I just said, this is a blood thinner. If I give too much, I can make someone's blood really thin and they can bleed. So it has always been a guessing game for cardiologists, and we usually err on the side of being conservative, where we say, "Let's start with a slightly lower dose, and see how you respond." But we do not have to do that anymore. Depending on an individual's genetic variants, they will be rapid or slow metabolizers of the drug. A rapid metabolizer obviously needs more.

We all have an example of this that we see in our friends and in our family which is caffeine. Some people can say, "Give me a triple espresso, and I am going to go to bed." And some of us look at that person and say, "How can you go to bed after a triple espresso?" Well that individual is most likely a rapid metabolizer of caffeine. Other individuals might say, "I can't even handle one cup of caffeine, it is just too much." So the genetic variants explain more than 50 percent of the variability in the requirement of Coumadin. And again, as I said before, this is important, because if someone is a rapid metabolizer, I can go ahead and give a slightly higher amount, but a slow metabolizer I want to start with a lower and safer dose.

I see a lot of women in my cardiology practice, and one question I get quite a bit is, "Should I be on aspirin?" And there are some guidelines for aspirin recommendations that we have, and of course, someone who has had a heart attack or has risk factors for heart disease like high blood pressure, we would say, "Yes, you should probably be on an aspirin." But there is now an interesting test called the LPA genotype test. We know that a single protein switch in this gene is associated with a higher risk of cardiac events and coronary artery disease.

We got some insight about this gene from a very important study called the Women's Health Initiative. What they found was this: If you give an aspirin to a non-carrier of the LPA variant (someone who does not have this little protein switch) it had no effect on reducing cardiovascular events. But in women who carried one copy of this risk variant, those women were at much higher risk for cardiovascular events, almost twice that of non-carriers. Why is it important? Because the women with this genetic variant, if we give them an aspirin, their risk is decreased, so if a woman has this genetic variant, I am going to say, "I want to recommend aspirin."

A couple of other questions come up in cardiology. One is, "Should I take statin therapy?" Statins are the drugs that lower cholesterol. And I just want to mention briefly that there is also a genetic test that can tell you whether or not you are prone to have a problem with metabolism of statins. What does that mean? Certain people in the population, when they take a statin cholesterol-lowering drug, they get muscle aches, joint aches, and pain. We now have a blood test that we can do to determine if you are at genetic risk for this problem. Obviously, if you are, then we want to try other medications that are not statin therapy.

Today we have discussed some of the fascinating research on the human genome. We have explored the new fields of nutrigenomics and pharmacogenomics. I really believe the big hope that these fields hold for the future. Even more importantly, we have seen that it is possible to turn genes on and off through nutrition and lifestyle change. That's where the science of natural healing comes in. In the rest of this course, you will be given the tools to make nutrition and lifestyle choices that can have positive and profound impact on your genes.

Food Matters
Lecture 4

With the right food, we do not need medicine. Food is medicine because food is information, and what we eat can have profound effects on our physical body. The right foods send a signal to our genes to produce a protein that prevents heart disease, Alzheimer's disease, arthritis, and inflammation, or we can choose to eat the wrong foods—those that are high in white refined flour and sugar—sending a signal to our genes to produce proteins that result in arthritis, back pain, shoulder pain, heart disease, and memory loss.

The China Study
- The China Study, which was conducted by T. Colin Campbell, analyzed 50 diseases in rural China and compared the food in China with the food in the United States to attempt to explain the diseases.
  - Fat intake was twice as high in the United States as it was in China.

  - The intake of fiber, which is found in fruits and vegetables, was three times lower in the United States.

  - The consumption of animal protein—such as beef, pork, and lamb—was 90 percent higher in the United States.

  - Heart disease death rates were 16 times greater in the United States for men and five times greater for women in comparison to rural China.

  - In the United States, cancer, osteoporosis, diabetes, and high blood pressure were more prevalent than in rural China.

- Campbell's study shows that food is linked to positive and negative health outcomes and that what we eat matters.

The Science of Nutrition

- Cardiologists know that some foods can impact the ability of blood vessels to dilate. The fat in a high-fat meal gets broken down into large particles that float around the bloodstream and can block blood vessels. A high-fat meal keeps a blood vessel from dilating for as long as six hours.

- If you lower the amount of fat in someone's diet, you improve the blood flow to his or her heart muscle. On the other hand, if you take someone with good blood flow and place him or her on a diet involving large quantities of saturated fats—a diet of beef, pork, and lamb, for example—the blood flow to the heart muscle is diminished.

- Research repeatedly links red meat, processed meat, and cured meat to colon cancer. In a study that was conducted by the National Institutes of Health (NIH) in 2010, over 3,000 Americans between the ages of 50 and 71 were analyzed. The NIH identified about 2,700 cases of colon cancer and concluded that red meat and processed meat are positively associated with colorectal cancer.

- Research that was conducted in 2010 shows that women who eat meat—particularly red and cured meat—prior to their diagnosis of ovarian cancer have a disadvantage in their clinical outcome.

- There are also links between obesity and cancer. There are about 100,000 deaths per year from cancer that are related to being overweight, and that is related to having too much sugar and simple carbohydrates in the diet.

- The good news is that there is also a lot of research on the positive influence of food that tells us what we should be eating, how we should be eating, and how much we should be eating.

- The *Archives of Internal Medicine* has shown that whole fruits and vegetables—particularly green leafy vegetables—protect against heart disease and stroke. Green leafy vegetables are high in calcium and magnesium and are very low in sugar.

- Research has shown that we can improve blood flow to the heart muscle with just lifestyle changes, such as diet, exercise, and support groups. In fact, plaque in vessels can be reversed in certain patients. They can turn on the right types of good proteins, such as the good HDL, and pull plaque out of their arteries.

The Mediterranean Diet
- The Mediterranean diet has gotten a lot of press over time because there are regions in the world where people do not have heart attacks. Epidemiologists conclude that the lack of heart attacks is related to the Mediterranean diet.

- Studies have shown that older people, 70 to 90 years of age, who follow a Mediterranean diet and simply walk about one mile per day enjoy a 50 percent lower rate of cardiac events and mortality.

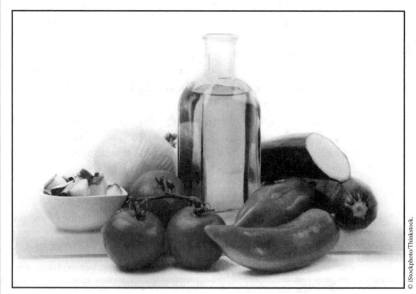

© iStockphoto/Thinkstock.

The Mediterranean diet focuses on healthy fats, fruits, and vegetables.

- The Mediterranean diet is associated with a reduction in cancer and cardiovascular events and an improvement in mortality from eating beans, lentils, legumes, whole foods, fruits, and fish. The Mediterranean diet is so effective because it is about the type of fats and carbohydrates in the diet.

- The carbohydrates that are consumed in the Mediterranean diet are whole grains, including whole wheat bread and brown rice.

- There are two kinds of fats that are important. Polyunsaturated fats include omega-6 and omega-3, and monounsaturated fats include olive oil and nuts.

- In the Mediterranean diet, people are told to stay away from saturated fats, such as beef, pork, lamb, lard, cream, and butter. They are told to use canola oil, which is monounsaturated, and they are told to eat a lot of omega-3s, which are polyunsaturated.

- When you eat omega-3s, particularly in the form of fish, you are going to send a signal to your genes that is going to produce proteins that prevent blood from clotting and block inflammation—which is linked to heart disease, Alzheimer's disease, and arthritis. This is one of the key ingredients of the Mediterranean diet's success.

- Think about your food as medicine. Every day, you should look at what you are eating and possibly keep a food journal or diary.

- Take your dinner plate and split it in half. Fill half of your plate with something green, such as green leafy vegetables, broccoli, asparagus, or escarole. Then, take the other half of your plate and divide it in half again. One half of that should be filled with whole grains, such as brown rice, wild rice, beans, and lentils. On the small quarter of a plate that is left, include good fats, such as a handful of nuts, a tablespoon of nut butter, some olive oil, or a small piece of avocado. Then, pick your protein, such as tofu, wild salmon, or an omega-3 powerhouse food.

- SMASH is an acronym for foods that are high in omega-3: sardines, mackerel, anchovies, salmon, and herring.

Questions to Consider

1. What research supports the role of nutrition in the prevention of cardiovascular disease?

2. What does "food is information" mean?

Food Matters
Lecture 4—Transcript

In Lecture 2, we talked about getting to the underlying cause of the problem, as one of the key principals for holistic integrative medicine. When I got to think about that as the physician, and I was conducting the research that I discussed, I had to teach myself something about food. Because remember, I was supposed to teach heart patients how to become vegetarian.

Let me tell you a true story. I drew my blood just like I drew my patients' blood, and I ran my own cholesterol level. And I was shocked. I could not believe it. I have always been thin, not that that makes a difference. I found that my cholesterol level was 320, and I thought, "Oh my God, I am going to die of heart disease." Of course, we know it is more than just about cholesterol, but that has sent me on a journey of learning everything I can about nutrition and how we can use nutrition for health. One of the key roots to our tree is micro and macro nutrition.

Hippocrates had it right. Hippocrates said, "Food is medicine." Why didn't we listen to him? If you look in Ayurvedic medicine, again, medicine that comes from India, they have a proverb that says, "With the right food, medicine is of no need. With the wrong food, medicine is of no use." Is that not fascinating?

So the wisdom of the ancients is telling us something about food. We also have the science today to take it to another level. We have now validated what Hippocrates is saying. If Hippocrates is saying food is medicine, we now have research that shows us why, because food is actually information.

What that tells us is that what we eat can have profound effects on our physical body. Let's take a look at a study that was done a number of years ago, but is still getting attention today. It is Campbell's work called, "The China Project." What he did was ask a simple question. He said, "Let's take a look at 50 diseases in rural China, and let's compare them to the United States, and let's see if we can learn something about the food in China versus the United States that can explain diseases." This is what he found. First, fat intake was twice as high in the United States. Of course, we know this, when we have a plate, it frequently has a steak on half the plate, if not three quarters of the plate. Fiber—and that is our fruits and our vegetables as you will see in a few minutes, legumes—our fiber intake in the United States was three times lower. Animal protein—beef, pork, lamb—90 percent higher in the United States. So they said, "Can we take these differences in the diet and look at trends in disease?" And this is what they found. Heart disease death rates are 16-fold greater in the United States for men, and 5-fold greater for women in the United States, in comparison to rural China. But it did not stop at heart disease, because as you will learn, as these lectures progress, what protects the heart, protects the bones from osteoporosis, protects from diabetes, high blood pressure, and cancer. So it was no surprise to me that in the United States we had more cancer, more osteoporosis, more diabetes, and more high blood pressure than in rural China. Just stop and think about it for a minute. I have been to rural China on a couple of occasions, and when you get a bowl of food, it is filled with green vegetables. I know everyone is thinking bok choy and things like that, and that would be right. For those that eat meat, meat on top is a garnish; it is not taking up three quarters of the plate.

What can we learn from Campbell's study? What kind of information does it give us? Well, it tells us that food is linked to positive and negative health outcomes. It tells us what we eat matters. Just like Hippocrates said, "Food is medicine." With the right food, we do not need medicine. Today, we are going to take a big look at some of the research that helps us understand this concept that food matters. Because my goal is to show you that there is science behind nutrition, and the nutrition recommendations that we will be going to make throughout this course.

I have a colleague named Dr. Vogel, and he is a great cardiologist. He likes to do a lot of experiments. In one of them, he puts a blood pressure cuff on the arm, and he pumps it up, and then he looks at the body's ability to dilate the blood vessel when the cuff is released. We have a term for this. It is called looking at endothelium-derived relaxation. Well, we do not need to know all that. All we know is that foods can impact the ability of our blood vessels to dilate. What he did was he had people come into his office and eat a high-fat meal. Now, I already knew high-fat meals were a problem, as a cardiologist, because this is what I would hear in my practice, "Hey Dr. G., we went to the restaurant, I had a big meal, I got up, and I was walking to the parking lot and all of the sudden I got chest pain, I had to stop and take a nitroglycerine." Why does that occur? It occurs because the fat in the meal get broken down into what we call BLDL, big particles that just float around the bloodstream, they can literally block blood vessels. But also what Vogel taught us is that the high fat meal keeps a blood vessel from dilating for as long as six hours. So think about that. Have you ever had a high-fat meal and you thought, "Why did I just do that? Why did I eat that?" because you do not feel good afterwards? Six hours, the ability of the blood vessels to the heart, now think about that, it is not getting blood flow for six hours at its maximum, just from the food.

One of the other areas I have to deal with in my practice is fad diets. Everyone wants to be on a particular type of named diet. Some people want to be really low fat, some people want to be really high fat and low carb, and so I said, "Let's take a look at the research. Let's take a look at what happens to blood flow to the heart when we take people and place them on a low-fat diet, and what happens to blood flow to the heart when we put people on a high fat diet." And this beautiful research was done by Dr. Fleming. What he did was look at blood flow scans to the heart muscle. This enables us to tell, are the arteries delivering enough blood to the regions of the heart? And what he found was this: If you take someone on a low-fat diet, you improve the blood flow to their heart muscle. If you lower the fat, you improve the blood flow. This is sort of what Ornish showed. What else did he show? He showed that if you take someone with good blood flow, this is really important, and you place them on a high saturated fat diet, beef, pork, lamb, gravy as a beverage, you know really high fat, the blood flow to the heart muscle is diminished.

For me as a cardiologist, that gives me a lot of information. That tells me, along with what I know about the inability of blood vessels to dilate, that the high-fat diet is not benefiting my heart patients.

Today the research is coming out over and over again that is linking red meat and processed meat, cured meats to colon cancer. One such study was conducted by the NIH, over 3000 Americans were looked at between the ages of 50 and 71. They identified about 2700 cases of colon cancer, and they concluded—this was done in 2010—that red meat and processed meat are positively associated with colorectal cancer. So it is not just a heart issue anymore, it is a cancer issue as well.

We have other very interesting research that has demonstrated the same thing. If you were to take a look at native Africans, and compare them to African-Americans—so two groups, native to Africa, those that have come here—what you would find is that the risk of colon cancer in a native African is one in 100,000, whereas the risk of colon cancer in an African-American is one in 2000. Now, there has to be a reason for this, and what this has been attributed to is animal protein, particularly the fat from red meat.

We also know that for women with ovarian cancer, and this is also recent, 2010, research shows us that women who eat meat prior to their diagnosis of ovarian cancer, particularly red and cured meat, have a disadvantage in their clinical outcome.

It is not only about the heart, it is about cancer, and as you will see in later lectures, we also have links now between obesity and cancer, we have about 100,000 deaths a year from cancer that are related to just being overweight, and we now know that that is related to too much sugar and simple carbohydrates in the diet.

I think it is pretty clear that diets high in red meat, which are inflammatory diets—and we will talk more about that later—and high in saturated fat, are linked to not only heart disease, but cancer as well. So the take home message is food matters. I tell my patients, "If your body is a Rolls Royce, what kind of gas do you want to put in your car?" and they say, "Well I have a Rolls Royce, I am going to put the most expensive gas." Well then why do we put junk food into our body? The good news is this: Just like I can cite research on the negative, we are going to spend some time talking about what we can do that makes a difference. The good news is we have as much research on the positive that tells us what we should be eating, how we should be eating, how much we should be eating, and so on. So on a good note, food does matter.

I can show lots of studies and of course I am only going to quote studies that are in major medical journals. Nothing is coming from the Journal of St. Elsewhere. From the *Archives of Internal Medicine* we learn that fruit and vegetables, whole fruits and vegetables, particularly green leafy vegetables, protect against heart disease. We also know that fruits and vegetables protect against stroke. And in a later lecture, we will be talking about specifically which ones. Green leafy vegetables are high in calcium, high in magnesium, very low in sugar, there is no sugar, does not spike up your insulin level, so no surprise to me that they protect against heart disease.

I mentioned in a previous lecture that I did some research with Dr. Dean Ornish and that is what led to my taking my own blood, starting to learn about nutrition, going to yoga class, and what we showed in that research was that we can improve blood flow to the heart muscle with just lifestyle change. Diet, exercise, vegetarian diet, and support groups. We actually were able to demonstrate in certain patients that we can reverse plaque in vessels. And I want to say that again, because a lot of patients ask me, "Can I reverse the plaque in my vessel?" and the answer is yes. We can turn on the right types of good proteins, like the good HDL, which you will learn more about, and pull plaque right out of the artery.

I thought about how I was raised, because I have a grandmother who came from Italy, and I was raised by my grandmother. I was not raised on packaged food. We always sat down for our meals, my grandmother prepared all the meals, the whole family came together for the meal, and as you will see later, that does make a difference. But it was what she served that I began to think about. Even though my grandmother was living in New York, in her mind, she was still in Calabria, Italy. She was serving the same foods. As a matter of fact, one of my grandmothers who came from Naples was growing all her own fruits and vegetables, and she was making wine in the basement. So I thought about what kind of food did we have on the table? Well we had lots of green things, things like escarole. My grandmother had a gallon of olive oil that was too heavy for me to pick up even today, and she would just put on the food. She was always sautéing garlic. She was always using rosemary. Basil everywhere, fresh tomatoes, salads. Yes, we had pasta, but not in huge amounts, small amounts of pasta. We had mushrooms and we had green beans. What she took with her from Italy back to New York was what everyone now calls the traditional Mediterranean diet.

This diet, over time, has gotten a lot of press because there are pockets, in Italy for example, where people do not have heart attacks. And yes, epidemiologists have gone in to study them, and at the end of the day, they always conclude the reduction in heart attacks, the lack of heart attacks, and so on is related to the Mediterranean diet. We have some studies that support this.

A very large trial was done looking at people who already had documented coronary disease. This was called the Lyon Diet Heart Study. It was a five-year trial. And it basically told people to eat the way my grandmother would have cooked for them, so they were told to eat more beans, eat more veggies, get their lentils in, they were told to use, in this particular study canola oil, but they certainly could have used olive oil. But they were asked to do something else: They were asked to eliminate saturated fat, beef, pork, and lamb. Hold it to a minimum. Eat more of the fish. They were asked to eliminate butter. They were asked to eliminate cream. Now we just heard how saturated fat is not good for the heart, not good for cancer. So what did they find? The study results were amazing. The Lyon Heart Study showed a 70 percent reduction in cardiovascular events. There is no drug on the market that can give us a 70 percent reduction in anything, and this is the Mediterranean diet. What was even more astounding is late cancers were reduced 80 percent. People developing cancer later in life was also reduced. So not only, again, were we helping the heart, which by the way if we help the heart, we help the brain, we help the kidneys, we help the bones and so on, but we were also preventing cancer.

We know that other research is telling us the same thing. Some of my patients come to me and say, "Dr. G., I am too old; I am too old to change. Will it make a difference in my life? I am 75." I say, "I want you to live 20 more years. I want you to live 20 more years. How do you want to live them? Do you want to live them with arthritis? Or do you want to have some health and vitality?" And you know that everyone always tells me health and vitality. So when other studies showed that if we take older people, 70 to 90 years of age, and they follow a Mediterranean diet, and they just simply walk one to 1.5 miles per day, 50 percent lower rate of cardiac events and mortality. Everything was affected in this study. This was called HALE Trial Project.

So we know that food matters. The research supports this. Why is this diet so effective? Why is the Mediterranean diet so effective? Reduction in cancer, reduction in cardiovascular events, and improvement in mortality from eating beans and lentils and legumes and whole foods and fruits and fish. Why is it so successful?

This is where modern day research comes in. Because we now know it is about the type of fat in the diet, and the type of carbohydrate in the diet. Now we will cover carbohydrates in a whole different lecture. But one thing my grandmother was not serving for dinner was white stuff. I was not eating white bread; I was only eating whole grain bread. My grandmother even made brown rice. And that is typical for the Mediterranean diet. There is not a lot of white stuff there. But it was also about the fat. There are two kinds of fats that are important to mention at this time. We call them polyunsaturated fats. That is our omega-6 and our omega-3. You hear this all the time, because people say, "I'm taking omega-3." Those are the polyunsaturated fats. And then we have monounsaturated fats, things like olive oil and nuts, and the Mediterranean diet, people were told stay away from your saturated fat, your beef, your pork, your lamb, your lard, your cream, your butter. They were told to use canola oil, mono unsaturated. And they were told to eat a lot of omega-3s.

What happens when we eat omega-3s, particularly in the form of fish? I said at the beginning of the talk, food is information, and here is a perfect example. If I decide that I am going to eat sardines, or I am going to eat a wild salmon, I am going to send a signal to my genes that is going to produce proteins that prevent blood from clotting and block inflammation. Inflammation is linked to heart disease, Alzheimer's disease, arthritis, everything you can think of. Just eating the omega-3s in the form of fish prevents the inflammation. We think that that is one of the key ingredients for the Mediterranean diet's success. Well, so does the American Medical Association. The American Medical Association had this to say, "Substantial evidence indicates that diets using non-hydrogenated fat" and we will talk about fats again throughout this course "whole grains as the main form of carbohydrates" and just as an aside, I tell my patients if you can roll your bread into a little ball, throw it out. I want real whole grain bread "an abundance of fruits and vegetables and adequate omega-3s can protect against heart disease." So this is what the *Journal of the American Medical Association* has to say. No hydrogenated fats, no trans-fats, no partially hydrogenated oils. Good fats, which we will talk about, like olive oil, like canola oil, like nuts, whole grains, like beans and lentils and legumes, fresh fruits and veggies, and omega-3s.

Well, I was really pleased, in 2009, to see another research article come out. Again, the *Journal of the American Medical Association* published an article saying, "Walking every day, physical activity, and eating a Mediterranean diet lowers the risk of Alzheimer's disease." Think about that. Now we have discussed cancer, heart disease, and now Alzheimer's disease. And I think you can probably see where I am going with this. There is really no disease, it is just mechanisms that lead to disease. We like to name them and place them in a silo, but what is good for the heart is good for the brain, and, by the way, it helps to prevent cancer.

I tell my patients I want them to think about their food as medicine. I want them, every day, to look at what they are eating. Sometimes I have them keep a food journal, or a food diary. I will ask them to write down everything on two week days and one weekend day, and then we will look at it together. I will ask them to take their dinner plate, a nice round dinner plate, and split it in half, and then I will tell them, "I want you to fill one half of that plate with something green—green leafy vegetables, broccoli, asparagus, escarole, all your greens, I want you to fill that half of the plate with." And then I tell them, "Take the other half of the plate and divide it in half, and one half of that is going to get your whole grains." And in this case I tell them, "Your brown rice, your wild rice, your beans, your lentils." We will talk more about this in the next lecture. And then on that little quarter of a plate that is left I say, "We have to include our good fats, so we have to start thinking about, do I have a handful of nuts, do I have a tablespoon of nut butter, do I have some olive oil, or a little piece of avocado?" Then I have them pick their protein, and the protein, which we will talk about again, can be something like tofu, or it could be wild salmon, or it can be an omega-3 powerhouse food. I will give you a little tip into the next lecture, we are going to learn an acronym which is SMASH, for our high-omega-3 foods, so the S is for sardines, the

M is for mackerel, the A is for anchovies, the second S is for salmon, good wild sockeye salmon, and the H is for herring.

At the end of the day, what we eat sends a signal to our genes to tell the gene to produce a protein that either prevents heart disease, prevents Alzheimer's disease, prevents arthritis, prevents inflammation. Or we can choose to eat the wrong foods, foods high in white refined flour, high in sugar, simple carbs, and that is going to send a signal to our genes that is going to produce proteins that, quite frankly, break us down, give us arthritis, give us back pain, give us shoulder pain, give us heart disease, and cause us to lose our memory.

Not All Foods Are Created Equal
Lecture 5

Research shows that food impacts our health, but not all foods are created equal. There are some unique properties of various foods that make them nutritional superstars. You should eat vegetables, grains, and legumes as whole foods; try not to process, refine, or filter them for the best effects. In addition, incorporate lean protein, preferably from the Earth, into your diet. Consume healthy forms of fat, such as olive oil, nuts, seeds, pumpkin, and flax. It is important to remember that how you cook a food can affect its nutritional content.

Whole Foods
- One of the nutrition superstars is whole foods, which are foods that are not processed, refined, or filtered.

- Whole foods are very high in phytonutrients, which mainly come from plants, vegetables, and fruits. They have beneficial effects on our body that are even greater than the effects of the vitamins, minerals, and micronutrients that we get when we eat a food.

- There are over 10,000 phytonutrients, which have antioxidant effects. They can boost the immune system and, therefore, prevent cancer. They are anti-inflammatory, and they can prevent heart disease and Alzheimer's disease. They are even antiviral and antibacterial; some of them behave like antibiotics. We typically find these foods in colored vegetables.

- The deeper the color of the food—the darker the berry or the redder the grape—the more phytonutrients it has. Vegetables, fruits, nuts, flax seeds, olive oil, and even chocolate are excellent sources of phytonutrients.

Refined Foods versus Whole Foods

- If the label on a particular type of food mentions that it is fortified with vitamins and minerals, that is actually a negative thing. Fortifying a food involves taking everything out of it. For example, if you take brown rice and decide to make white rice, you are stripping the rice of all of its good qualities.

- Refining food removes important vitamins and minerals. For example, 77 percent of thiamine, which can only be obtained through food, is removed; 76 percent of iron, which is needed to make red blood cells, is removed; 85 percent of magnesium, which is needed not only to keep our bowels moving but also to keep our heart healthy, is removed. When food is refined, copper, zinc, calcium, and everything that we need to have strong and healthy bones is also removed.

- One of the greatest things that whole foods give us is fiber. Soluble fiber is found in foods such as beans, peas, nuts, apples, and vegetables. Fiber is important in lowering cholesterol and blood sugar. It binds the fatty acids in the intestine and pulls them out of the body. Fiber also blocks the quick absorption of sugar.

- When adding fiber—ideally 35 grams per day—to your diet, a few categories are important.
    o Whole grains: Steel-cut oats are a perfect example of a whole grain, and psyllium is one of the most potent sources of soluble fiber.

    o Fruits: You should eat two to three whole fruits, including dark berries and apples, per day.

    o Legumes and beans: These carry a lot of fiber.

    o Vegetables: Green leafy vegetables have calcium and magnesium, do not have sugar, do not spike up your insulin, and contain lots of fiber.

- You have to gradually add fiber into your diet—especially if you are not used to eating it—because if you add a lot of fiber suddenly, you will experience a lot of gas and bloating.

Vegetables

- Broccoli contains sulforaphane, which is an anticancer food that eliminates toxins from our body.

- Green vegetables such as arugula, bok choy, brussels sprouts, mustard greens, kale, cauliflower, cabbage, collard greens, watercress, and radishes have similar effects to broccoli on your body.

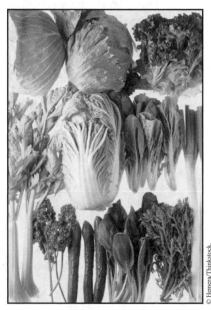

- Spinach is very high in antioxidant activity, and research shows that it is good for the eyes.

- Mushrooms, such as shitake, maitake, enoki, and oyster mushrooms, are medicinal. However, those small white button mushrooms can actually contain toxins. For best results, sauté your mushrooms in turmeric.

© Hemera/Thinkstock.

- Lycopene occurs in tomatoes and can prevent prostate cancer. It can even lower blood pressure and block platelets from sticking together, which is the first step to having a heart attack.

Green vegetables that turn on the same enzymes in your body as broccoli include cauliflower, cabbage, and collard greens.

Berries

- Blueberries contain anthocyanosides, which protect the eye, give you the most potent antioxidant that is good for your heart, and block bacteria from sticking to the lining of your bladder.

- Ingesting cranberry is actually like taking an antibiotic. It contains hippuric acid, and just like the blueberry, it blocks *E. coli*—one of the most common pathogens for urinary tract infections—from sticking to the lining of the bladder.

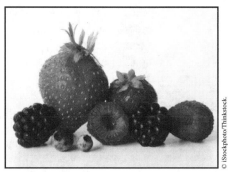

Buy berries that have thin skins—such as strawberries, blueberries, raspberries, and blackberries—organic.

Nuts

- Nuts are a source of fiber and protein. They also contain magnesium, zinc, calcium, and vitamin E—an antioxidant.

- Walnuts have over 16 polyphenols, which are phytonutrients with strong antioxidant ability. They help to protect our heart and brain.

- Do not eat too many nuts because they have a lot of calories. Instead, use them as a garnish; for example, put them on top of a salad.

Fats and Proteins

- Saturated fats are solid at room temperature and are found in beef, lard, cream, cheese, and butter.

- Unsaturated fats contain two categories. Monounsaturated fats typically come from the Earth and are found in olives, nuts, and seeds. Polyunsaturated fats contain two main groups: Omega-6s comes from corn, corn oil, safflower oil, and sunflower oil, and omega-3s come from fish.

- The ideal omega-6 to omega-3 ratio is two to one. Olive oil has a ratio of around 13 to one, which is great for an oil. Avocado oil is even better for cooking than olive oil because you can cook avocado oil at high temperatures, but olive oil becomes toxic at high temperatures. The perfect oil is macadamia nut oil, which has a ratio of one to one. It also has a slightly higher heating point, so it can be used for cooking.

- Proteins that come from the Earth are things like edamame, nuts, and legumes. Proteins that come from animals are omega-3 eggs, low-fat yogurt, fish, chicken, and turkey.

Cooking Matters
- The way we prepare a food can lead to the production of bad chemicals, such as lipid peroxidases, advanced glycation end products (AGEs), and heterocyclic amines.

- AGEs make proteins more likely to rev up our immune system. They lead to inflammation, accelerate aging, and make heart disease and brain disease much worse.

- We ingest AGEs by cooking in high temperatures, and we inhibit them by cooking with moisture. When you can, boil your food for only a few minutes, poach, and use a steamer. The more you fry, broil, and roast, the more you increase the AGEs in your food.

Questions to Consider

1. Which fats are monounsaturated and polysaturated?

2. What is a phytonutrient?

Not All Foods Are Created Equal
Lecture 5—Transcript

In the previous lecture we had a long discussion about some of the research looking at how food impacts our health. We concluded beyond a shadow of a doubt that food matters. And as I tell my patients, "food first." But not all food is created equally. There are some unique properties of different foods that make them what I like to call nutrition superstars.

Let's get started. The first nutrition superstar is whole foods. Now, many of my patients look at me when I say, "I want you to eat whole foods. I want you to eat real food." What do I mean by that? I do not want your food to be processed, to be refined, I do not even want it to go past a filter and be juiced. I want you to eat the whole apple. I want you to eat the whole grain, the whole bean, and the whole vegetable. Just the way the Earth gives it to us: whole.

Why do I want you to eat whole foods? Because whole foods are very high in something called phytonutrients. Phytonutrients come from plants, and they come from vegetables, and fruits, and we even see them in other foods as well. They have beneficial effects on our body. And these effects are even above the vitamins, the minerals, and the micronutrients that we get when we eat a food. There are over 10,000 phytonutrients. They have antioxidant effects. They can boost the immune system, and therefore prevent cancer. They are anti-inflammatory. They can prevent heart disease and Alzheimer's disease. They are even antiviral, antibacterial. Some of them actually behave like antibiotics. We typically find these foods in colored vegetables.

The deeper the color, the darker the berry, the redder the grape, the more phytonutrients it has. We find them in vegetables, we find them in fruits, but we also find them in my favorite food: chocolate. And we will talk a little bit about that in another lecture. But nuts, flax seeds, even olive oil are excellent sources as well.

What happens when we refine a food? You may notice on a breakfast cereal box that it says, "fortified with vitamins and minerals." Well, that word fortified is one of my red flags, because if we have to fortify a food, that means we took everything out of it. For example, if we take brown rice and we decide to make white rice, we are stripping the rice of all its good stuff. Refining foods remove important vitamins and minerals. For example, 77 percent of thiamine is removed from a refined food. You can only get thiamine from food. You can't get it in any other way unless you take a supplement. And refined foods strip it right out. Iron, 76 percent is removed. I know this audience knows that iron is needed to make red blood cells. And my favorite mineral, magnesium, magnesium is needed not only to keep our bowels moving, but the heart loves magnesium, it prevents extra heartbeats, skipped heartbeats, what we call, in cardiology, arrhythmia, 85 percent of the magnesium is removed from refined foods. What about our bones? When we refine the food, we pull out copper, zinc, calcium, everything that we need to have strong and healthy bones. And this is just a little bit of the list.

One of the greatest things that whole foods give us is fiber. Why do we need fiber? Fiber is like a miracle food. Soluble fiber, which we find in foods like beans and peas, even nuts and apples, all of our vegetables, fiber is so important in lowering cholesterol and in lowering blood sugar. I have patients in my practice that can't take statin medications for their cholesterol. The first thing I tell them is, "Every morning, I want you to make steel-cut oats." I see drops in cholesterol from 50 to 70 points just adding fiber to the diet. How does it work? Fiber binds the fatty acids right in the intestine and pulls them out of the body. It also blocks the quick absorption of sugar. Let me give you an example. When we eat a whole food, when we eat an apple, we do get sugar (an apple has natural sugar). But we also get the fiber from the apple, so when we eat the whole apple, the fiber slows down the absorption of the sugar from the apple, therefore we do not spike up our insulin level—insulin leads to inflammation, it puts weight on in our midline, insulin is a really bad player for us. If we decide, "Let's take that apple and make apple juice," and we run that apple through a series of filters and we come out with apple juice, and we drink the apple juice—guess what?—we have removed all of the fiber. And by removing the fiber, the juice goes right into our bloodstream, the body sees it as sugar, sugar, sugar, sugar, turn on the insulin, we turn on the insulin and all of the sudden we get high for a few minutes, and then the insulin drops our blood sugar back down. So we want to use the whole food with the fiber.

It may even end up being a treatment for prostate cancer. And, it has some other added benefits. It can even lower blood pressure, and block the platelets from sticking together—which, by the way, is the first step to having a heart attack, sticky platelets. So add some lycopene in, slice up some tomatoes. But what I do not want you to do, if you tend to have heartburn for example, don't go and make a lot of red tomato sauce, because that can really make heartburn worse.

Let's move on to another category. Let's take a look at some of the berries. You remember when I talked about phytonutrients, I mentioned berries, and I said the darker the berry or the darker the grape, the more phytonutrients it has. Probably one of the key berries is the blueberry. Blueberries contain something called anthocyanosides. Basically what that translates into is there is a component of the blueberry that protects the eye. So again, just like we talked about earlier with the spinach, adding blueberries into your diet not only gives you the most potent antioxidant which is good for your heart, but it also is giving you something special for your eyes, and a third thing that blueberries can do, they can actually block bacteria from sticking to the lining of your bladder. So when I see women in my practice that say. "You know Dr. G., I get those urinary tract infections all the time." I say, "Let's add some whole blueberries, organic, to your diet, and let's also add my second favorite berry, the cranberry." Cranberry is actually like taking an antibiotic. It has something called hippuric acid. And just like the blueberry, it blocks *E. coli*, one of the common pathogens for urinary tract infections from sticking to the lining of the bladder. Those are some of the superstars. There are many. This is just the tip of the iceberg.

We talked about fiber, and we said we get our fiber from our fruits and our vegetables, our whole grains, our oats, our steel-cut oatmeal, and our beans. But we also get fiber from another source. We can also get it from nuts. And I mentioned in a previous lecture that I have been a vegetarian for many years, so as a vegetarian, I have to incorporate nuts as a source of protein in my diet. Nuts have lots of wonderful properties. They contain micronutrients, magnesium, which I mentioned is good for the heart, zinc, and calcium, which we talked about being good for the bones. They also have vitamin E, which is an antioxidant, protects the brain, protects the heart, and they have fiber. If we have to have a king of the nuts, we would have the walnut.

The walnut has over 16 polyphenols. These are phytonutrients with strong antioxidant ability, they protect our heart, they protect our brain.

There is one caveat about nuts: You can eat them, but don't eat too many. I tell my patients don't go to some big store and buy a big thing of nuts like this and eat the whole thing—especially while you are watching TV—because nuts have a lot of calories. So if you have, for example, 10 walnut halves, or you have maybe 15 or 20 almonds, or 15 or so cashews, you are getting about 180 calories. So that is a lot of calories, but it is good calories. How do I want you to use nuts? I want you to use them as a garnish. Put them on top of your salad. This morning for breakfast I had steel-cut oats and I put walnuts, the king of the nut, on top of my oatmeal. That is how I want you to use them. I also will take nuts like almonds and I will make my broccoli, just blanch it quickly in a little bit of water, I will add some turmeric and some garlic and then put some nuts on top and that is really a perfect food.

One of the common questions I get from my patients is, "Hey Dr. G., do I have to buy organic? Does everything have to be organic? It is a little bit more expensive; I can't afford it." And this is how I teach it to my patients. I say, "If you buy organic, you are not getting the fertilizers that are chemical fertilizers. You are getting natural fertilizers. You are not getting anywhere up to 450 pesticides." Do you know that non-organic strawberries have been sprayed over 30 times before they get to your supermarket? You also are not getting hormones and antibiotics, you are getting crop rotation, meaning the soil, the organic soil has all of the micronutrients that we need, so I tell my patients, "Sorry, but I prefer you to buy organic."

If someone wants to buy nonorganic, I say, "Okay. Let's go after the ones that are really a problem." That means the dirty dozen. And you can go to a website called *The Environmental Working Group*, and they list the dirty dozen, they change it all the time, they are monitoring the food. But the way I think about it is this way. If it has a thin skin, a strawberry, a berry, an apple, a peach, a pear, a plum, I want it organic. If I can peel it, and it has a thick skin, like an onion, or an avocado, or a mango, or a pineapple, I am a little less worried about it being organic.

We talked a lot about fruits and vegetables, and we have to think about our dinner plate again. If half of our dinner plate is our green leafy vegetables, and we are having our three whole fruits a day, and a quarter of our dinner plate is our whole grains, our wild rice, our beans, our lentils, we have to decide about our protein, and we also have to decide about our fat. This is an area where I see a lot of confusion. There is so much confusion about fat. So let's take a minute to walk through the different kinds of fats.

Saturated fats are solid at room temperature. They are the kinds of fats like beef, lard, cream, even cheese. These are saturated fats. Butter is an example of a saturated fat. It is solid at room temperature.

Then we have something called unsaturated fats. And there are two big categories; this is the way I like to remember it. Monounsaturated fats typically come from the Earth. They are things like our olives, so our olive oil, our nuts, our seeds. Those are all monounsaturated.

And then, this is where it gets a little tricky. We have polyunsaturated. And there are two big groups here: the omega-3s and the omega-6. Omega-6 comes from corn, corn oil, safflower oil, sunflower oil, and a few others. The omega-3s we have talked about. They come from fish. Remember we talked about sockeye salmon, sardines, mackerel, anchovy, herring? That is where we get our omega-3s. Now why is it important?

In the first nutrition talk I mentioned a concept, that food is information. The ideal omega-6 to omega-3 ratio is two to one. The typical American diet is 20 to one or 50 to one, depending on what you are eating. Don't worry about getting your omega-6s; it's everywhere. You have to worry about getting enough omega-3. Why? Because when you eat omega-3, when you decide, "I'm having that wild sockeye salmon, I'm having those sardines," and we will talk about omega-3 supplements, you are turning on genes that are anti-inflammatory. You produce proteins that protect you against heart disease, Alzheimer's disease, and cancer. So we want to have a good dose of omega-3s because the more omega-6 we have, the more disease we have.

Where do we go? What kind of fats do we eat? Well, I like olive oil. Olive oil has an omega-6 to omega-3 ratio of around 13 to one. That is one of the best for an oil. Avocado oil is another option. And it is even better for cooking than olive oil. Olive oil can't be cooked under high temperatures, do not boil your olive oil, do not cook olive oil in a high flame; it becomes toxic. If you are going to cook in high temperatures, use avocado oil. And of course the perfect oil is the macadamia nut oil. Get this: This oil has an omega-6 to omega-3 ratio of one to one. It is perfect. It also has a slightly higher heating point, so it can be used for cooking. I still like to use the avocado oil and very rarely for high temperatures, a little bit of coconut oil. Small amounts, remember oil has a lot of calories.

Let's go to one other very big category. The last thing on our plate is protein. What kind of protein do we eat? The hardest thing to me when I became a vegetarian was finding protein. I always thought of protein as beef, pork, and lamb, things like that. Well, I teach my patients that you can have protein from the Earth or protein from animals. Proteins from the Earth are things like edamame, nuts, and legumes. Proteins from animals are omega-3 eggs, low-fat yogurt, fish, chicken, and turkey. This comes up a lot in my practice. People will say, "Dr. G., I have kidney problems, I can't eat protein." We don't want you to eat animal protein when you have kidney problems—we're not worried about the vegetable protein; it's the animal protein that puts a stress on the kidneys.

Let's go through a series of our healthy choices. We have already talked about green leafy vegetables. There are some things you can eat unlimited amounts of, things like artichokes, asparagus, bamboo shoots, bell peppers (remember those have to be organic), broccoli, cabbage, cauliflower, turns on those phase II enzymes, okra, onions, summer squash, zucchini, eat these without limitation. Also bring in more greens—the more kale you can do, the more escarole, the more Swiss chard, spinach we talked about, dandelion, and arugula—this is all power food. These are your nutrition superstars. Have your three whole fruits a day. Make it a low-sugar fruit, apples, cherry, peach, pear, plum, go for those dark berries, they are perfect, even an orange or a grapefruit.

What about nuts? Remember, use them as a garnish, add the almonds on top, add the walnuts, cashews, pecans, and even seeds—sunflower seeds and pumpkin seeds. Make your grains whole grain. If you can roll your bread into a little ball I tell my patients "Throw it out." We want you to have real grains, brown rice. White rice is out. We do not want that. Quinoa is in. Bulgur is in. Legumes—plenty of them—lentils, beans, lima beans, kidney beans. The most digestible bean there is is something called the mung bean. And make edamame; snack on some edamame. It is a great snack, it is the soy bean, you just blanch it in a little bit of warm water, you can put some turmeric on top, and you have a perfect snack food.

Protein, remember SMASH, those are our good fish. We have our omega-3 eggs. Why do I want the omega-3? Because the ratio of the omega-6 to omega-3 is better in those eggs. Organic yogurts, tofu, tempeh, beans, lentils, are all good choices. And use the olive oil, or you can use canola oil. We didn't mention that one, but you can. You can use avocado oil, macadamia oil, small amounts of seeds, olives, nuts, a tablespoon of nut butter, remember these are good fats, but just like nuts, they are fattening.

I just want to touch on one other area before we close this lecture. And that is on cooking. I never really thought about how cooking matters. If food matters, cooking matters. The way we prepare a food can lead to the production of really bad chemicals. Something called lipid peroxidases, advanced glycation end products, heterocyclic amines—these sound terrible, I do not want to eat them, and I can get them just by preparing food in the wrong way.

Let's take a look at the advanced glycation end products (AGEs). These guys make proteins more likely to rev up our immune system. They lead to inflammation. They accelerate aging. And they make heart disease much worse, brain disease much worse. They totally rev up the inflammatory response. So how do we get them? We get these AGEs by cooking in high temperature. And we inhibit them by cooking with moisture. So I tell all my patients boil for a few minutes when you can, poach when you can, by a steamer, a bamboo steamer is a perfect way to go. Because the more we fry, broil—and I know no one's going to deep fry here—and the more we roast (so fry, broil, and roast) we increase the AGEs in our food.

Let's take a look at three ounces of chicken. If we oven fry it, it has 9000 AGEs. If we boil it, it is 1000. And if we roast it, it is about 4000 or so, half the amount of oven-fried.

So in conclusion, there are four things I want you to remember. First: whole foods, mainly vegetables, grains, and legumes. Second: lean protein, preferably from the Earth. Third: healthy forms of fat, olive oil, nuts, seeds, pumpkin, and flax. And last but not least, how you cook a food can affect its nutrition content.

Natural Approaches to Inflammation
Lecture 6

The foods that we eat can lead to, or prevent, inflammation, which is one of the final pathways for most of the common diseases. Inflammation is a crucial protective reaction; it is there to protect us so that healing can take place. In this lecture, you will learn some of the main causes of chronic inflammation. More importantly, you will learn how you can reverse the process—and even prevent it in the first place—by understanding the underlying causes.

Causes of Inflammation

- Inflammation is our body's normal response to an injury, an infection, stress, foreign substances, and anything that might be irritating us.

- In medicine, we use the suffix "-itis" to mean "inflammation"—for example, pharyngitis is an inflammation of the throat, or sore throat. The classic signs of inflammation are swelling, redness, pain, and warmth. The body turns on its defense mechanism to defend against a toxin or foreign invader.

- Cancer, Alzheimer's disease, and heart disease are all linked to inflammation. In fact, most cardiologists today are less worried about cholesterol as it relates to blockage in the arteries than about inflammation. Inflammation is more important.

- Polluted air, chemical irritants, second-hand smoke, and pesticides are all seen by the body as foreign invaders. They turn on our immune system; they are foreign particles that the body is responding to. This irritation can lead to chronic inflammation of the lung and can even increase the risk of cancer.

- Ulcers are chronic infections that are caused by a bacterium called *Helicobacter pylori*. This bacterium sits in the stomach, produces inflammation, can cause ulcers, and can even cause stomach cancer.

- A sensitivity or allergy to a food causes an inflammatory response. An allergy is a quick reaction, and the immune response is that we produce a protein called IGE. A food sensitivity has a more gradual course that leads to chronic low-grade inflammation, and it involves an immune factor called IGG.

- Another common cause of inflammation is midline weight, which involves wearing your weight around the midline of your body. Those fat cells are actually an inflammatory organ, and they produce cytokines, which raise blood pressure, cause inflammation, and make a person diabetic.

- If you have chronic sleep disturbance or even just a few hours of lost sleep, the body turns on its defense system, which leads to inflammation.

- Sleep apnea affects those who snore and then stop breathing. This can also lead to chronic inflammation and weight gain.

Food and Inflammation

- What you eat can turn inflammation on, but more importantly, what you eat can turn inflammation off.

- There are eight major foods that contribute to inflammation.
  - The number one cause of inflammation is sugar, which exists in the form of corn syrup, dextrose, fructose, golden syrup, maltose, and sucrose. If you have any signs of inflammation or any problems linked to inflammation—such as heart disease, memory loss, and arthritis—eliminate sugar.

  - There are good oils that have a very good omega-6 to omega-3 ratio, and then there are oils that are very high in omega-6. Stand clear of oils that are high in omega-6, such as grape-seed oil, cottonseed oil, corn oil, safflower oil, and sunflower oil. These are industrial vegetable oils that are usually found in fast foods and processed foods.

o   Trans fats are a modified form of fat that increase and oxidize the bad cholesterol, or LDL, which leads to the laying down of plaque in the vessel. They also lower the good cholesterol, or HDL. Trans fats are found in deep-fried foods, fast foods, and commercially prepared baked goods, and they usually appear on labels as "partially hydrogenated oil."

o   Cow's milk also leads to inflammation. People who are lactose intolerant typically develop stomach distress, diarrhea, gas, and bloating, but milk is also a common cause of arthritis and skin rashes.

o   Cured meats and red meats contain a substance called neu5Gc, which is a compound that the body sees as a foreign invader, so it produces antibodies and triggers an inflammatory response.

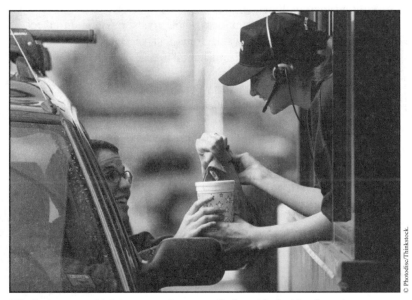

Oils that are very high in omega-6 are usually found in fast foods and processed foods.

     o   Excess alcohol consumption is rampant in our culture and is linked to irritation and inflammation of the esophagus. Esophageal and laryngeal cancers are linked to alcohol consumption. High consumption of alcohol affects the liver as well—from cirrhosis to alcohol-induced hepatitis. Over time, chronic inflammation from alcohol can lead to tumor progression.

     o   Another cause of inflammation is the consumption of refined grains, such as white bread and white rice. Do not eat anything white.

     o   Artificial food additives, such as monosodium glutamate and aspartame trigger the inflammatory response. Do not buy anything in a package unless you can read the label and identify all of the ingredients.

Preventing Inflammation

- To prevent inflammation, eat whole foods: fish high in omega-3, kelp (seaweed), and whole fruits and vegetables. Use olive oil, avocado oil, and macadamia nut oil instead of oil made from corn.

- Drink filtered water, but do not drink water from plastic bottles because it is not good for the environment—or for your health.

- Tea is the second-most consumed beverage in the world next to water. Research on black tea shows that black tea dilates blood vessels, which is a good thing. Like broccoli, turmeric, and shitake mushrooms, green tea can protect against cancer. It is anti-inflammatory and can reduce cardiovascular disease.

- Herbs and spices, when used correctly, have powerful anti-inflammatory components.

- Tulsi, also called holy basil, is an Ayurvedic herb that comes from India and is pure anti-inflammatory.

- Turmeric contains a powerful nontoxic compound called curcumin, which is what makes mustard have a yellow color. Research studies have shown that turmeric is as good, on occasion, as hydrocortisone and Motrin for inflammation. Turmeric also has anticancer properties.

- Ginger is a spice that has powerful anti-inflammatory benefits. It also has the added benefit of helping with nausea—not only related to cancer and chemotherapy, but also related to pregnancy.

- Basil, which is a staple in the Italian diet, is anti-inflammatory—as is rosemary.

Questions to Consider

1. What are three causes of inflammation?

2. Name three anti-inflammatory foods.

Natural Approaches to Inflammation
Lecture 6—Transcript

In the previous lecture we discussed that not all foods are created equally. We concluded again that food matters, and that nutrition is a key component to our health.

As we have already seen the foods that we eat can lead to, or prevent, inflammation. And inflammation is one of the final common pathways for most of the diseases that I see every day in my practice.

The first question is: What is inflammation? And is it all bad? Well, it is not all bad, because inflammation is our body's normal response to an injury. It is a normal response to infection, to stress, to foreign substances, and anything that might be irritating us.

So, for example, in medicine we use the term -itis to mean inflammation. We say hepatitis, pharyngitis, inflammation of the throat, or sore throat. So when we have inflammation, we have swelling, we have redness, we have pain, we have warmth, these are the classic signs of inflammation. The body is turning on its defense mechanism to defend against some sort of toxin—or in the case of a pharyngitis, a foreign invader as we say.

It is a crucial protective reaction. It is there to protect us so that healing can take place.

But what if you have a chronic illness? What happens if you have inflammation in your gums? Around your teeth? Here comes the -itis again: gingivitis. What if you are under a lot of stress? Your body is constantly being exposed to what is called inflammatory cytokines. If you have inflammation in your gums, your body is constantly trying to fight that inflammation. How do I see it in my practice? People come in to see me and they say, "Hey, Dr. G., my joints hurt, I have shoulder pain, I have elbow pain, knee pain." They may have ulcers. They may have a classic form of inflammation called emphysema or asthma, irritation of the lung. They may have eczema, psoriasis, skin rashes. I also see, of course, heart disease, and inflammation of the colon. Something called colitis.

I also see the end result of inflammation. We see things like cancer now, linked to inflammation, Alzheimer's disease, and, as you will hear me talk about throughout these lectures, heart disease. As a matter of fact most cardiologists today are less worried about cholesterol as it relates to blockage in the arteries than worried about inflammation. Inflammation is more important.

Today we will review some of the causes of chronic inflammation. But what is even more important when we leave this lecture we will know what we can do to put the fire out. How can we reverse the process? We can get to the underlying cause as we have said in the beginning; we can reverse the inflammation and prevent it in the first place.

So what causes chronic inflammation? Well, one that you might not think about is polluted air or chemical irritants—particles in the air, second-hand smoke, pesticides. All of these the body sees, again, as foreign invaders. They turn on our immune system. They are foreign particles that the body is responding to. This irritation can lead to chronic inflammation of the lung. I have already mentioned asthma; possibly other parts of the body will be affected as well. And yes, it can even increase the risk of cancer.

I would like to take a minute to talk about one other common cause that most people do not think about. We are all used to having an infection and taking an antibiotic, and the bacteria gets cleared and we feel better. But what about chronic infections? We actually know that ulcers, peptic ulcer disease, are caused by a bacterium. It is called Helicobacter pylori. This bacteria sits in our stomach, produces inflammation, can cause ulcers, and can even cause stomach cancer. So if someone has Helicobacter pylori, you do not say, "Oh, let's just give you anti-acids," you want to treat the Helicobacter. One of the things that I see in my practice is people come in with lab results that are showing inflammation. And no one has bothered to check them for inflammation of the gums, what we call gingivitis. No one has bothered to question them about their stomach. Maybe it is this Helicobacter. And one of my favorites is food sensitivity.

Being sensitive or allergic to a food is so important that it is a topic all to itself in another lecture. But if we have a sensitivity, or an allergy, to a food, that sets up an inflammatory response. There is a difference between sensitivity and allergy, and we will be reviewing this throughout a few lectures. But just to make it really simple, an allergy is a quick reaction. I am allergic to peanuts; I eat a peanut and I may not be able to breathe. My body may swell up. I might get what we call edema. The immune response is that we produce a protein called IGE. The way I teach it to my patients, I say remember, IGE, the E is for emergency, that is what happens with an allergy. But what happens with a food sensitivity? Well, it has a slower, more gradual course that like the Helicobacter leads to chronic low-grade inflammation. This has a different immune factor involved with it. It is called IGG, G. as in George, or G. as in Gradual. So that is an easy way to remember them.

I have a story that is really worth telling here. I was asked to see a middle-aged man who was a corporate executive. He was actually dragged in by his wife, which, by the way in my practice is not an uncommon scenario. And he came in because he was having some chest discomfort, and his wife was concerned he had heart disease. But when I started to question him, he was getting injections every month in his butt with an antibiotic and a steroid. And I said, "I do not know of any medical condition that would warrant you having these injections every month." and he said to me, "Dr. G., if I do not take those injections, my joints are so bad I can't get out of bed in the morning. I can't even walk." He said "And then what happens? I get this horrible skin rash that everyone can see." He said, "I can't go into a board meeting covered in a skin rash, so every month, I have these injections." Well, what we did with him was we decided to test him, to do a genetic test for gluten. I was so convinced he had gluten sensitivity. So I brought this up to him and he said to me, "There is no way. That can't be right. I am not stopping my gluten." And I can tell you now, six years later, after stopping his gluten, not touching it again he has no symptoms, no need for antibiotics, and he has absolutely no need for steroids. He is now a believer.

And as I said earlier, this is so important we will spend a whole lecture on food sensitivity and food allergy. Let's go to another common cause of inflammation. I see this one also every day in my practice: It is midline weight—just wearing your weight in the midline—because those fat cells are actually an inflammatory organ. They are an endocrine organ, and they produce all sorts of what we call cytokines. These cytokines raise our blood pressure, cause inflammation, and make us diabetic. So just carrying that midline weight is a source of inflammation.

Another big one is lack of sleep. If you have chronic sleep disturbance or even just a few hours of lost sleep, the body says turn on the defenses, we have a problem here. And that defense system leads to inflammation. And there is one that is really worth mentioning at this time, which is something called sleep apnea, or sleep disorder breathing: people who snore and then stop breathing. This can also lead to chronic inflammation. It also leads to weight gain. And one of the most interesting articles that just came out this week has identified that lack of sleep results in people eating 500 more calories per day. And you might say why? Why do people eat more calories if they do not sleep? Because they are using the food during the day to perk themselves up. If I eat sugar, I will wake up, that is what people think.

So far we have discussed some of the main causes of inflammation. There are some genetic causes as well, but the big ones we have already hit on: environmental toxins, microorganisms, food sensitivity, carrying extra weight in the midline, and lack of sleep or even sleep apnea. I mentioned very briefly stress. Stress is so important that we have more than one lecture dedicated to that topic alone.

Let's turn to the biggest category: food. You have already heard me say what you eat can turn inflammation on, more importantly what you eat can turn inflammation off.

Let's take a quick look at the eight major foods that contribute to inflammation. This is a big one, sugar. Sugar is probably number one. And I know you are thinking, "Oh, but I eat brown sugar." No different. Sugar is the number one cause of inflammation and again, it is so important that we have an entire lecture dedicated to it. No matter what name it hides under, and these are just a few: corn syrup, dextrose, fructose, golden syrup—boy that sounds like it is healthy—maltose, and sucrose. It is still sugar, and it leads to inflammation. If you have any signs of inflammation, or any problems linked to inflammation like heart disease, memory loss, arthritis, just to name a few, the first thing I want you to do is eliminate sugar. As a matter of fact, I can't think of a good reason for you to be eating sugar right now, refined white sugar, no good reason.

Let's take a look at oils. I have mentioned oils in a previous lecture. So there are good oils that have a very good omega-6 to omega-3 ratio, and then there are oils that are very high in omega-6. I want you to stand clear of these oils. These include grape seed oil, cottonseed oil, corn oil, safflower oil, and sunflower oil. These are industrial vegetable oils. They are usually in fast foods and they are in processed foods. So, those oils we need to avoid.

You will hear a common term called trans-fats. Trans-fats are a modified form of fat that do a lot of bad things. First of all they increase our LDL, or our bad cholesterol, even more importantly they oxidize the LDL, and that oxidized LDL leads to the laying down of plaque in the vessel. They also lower the good cholesterol, what we call the HDL. Now, in the previous lecture you heard me say do not deep-fry your foods. There is no reason to deep-fry anything. Trans-fats are found in deep-fried foods, fast foods, commercially prepared baked goods, they are just added in. And they usually will appear on the label as partially hydrogenated oil. So when you look on your label I want you to avoid trans-fats.

You might be thinking, "Oh I know all this, this makes sense, I have heard trans-fats are bad," but the next one might surprise you.

The next one that leads to inflammation is milk. That is right, milk, cow's milk. Sixty percent of the world's population can't digest milk. In fact, researchers think that being able to digest milk beyond infancy is actually abnormal. Now, a lot of people know, "Gee, I can't drink milk, I am quote-unquote lactose intolerant," and what happens in that situation, they develop stomach distress, diarrhea, gas, bloating, what most people do not realize, milk is a common cause of arthritis and a common cause of skin rashes.

Another big category, one of my favorite, favorite topics, and this is something I do not think most people have heard is cured meats and red meat contain a substance called neu5Gc. This is a compound that the body sees, again, as a foreign invader. It produces antibodies to it and triggers an inflammatory response. So yes, red meat, again, we saw it implicated in colon cancer, worse prognosis in ovarian cancer, intimately linked to heart disease, and now I am telling you one of the common bases for that is inflammation.

The link between processed meat consumption and cancer is really strong. Commercially produced meats, animals living on feedlots, are fed soybeans and corn. Think about this for a second. Eating meat that is from an animal, which is high in omega-6, leads to inflammation. This is one of the things I tell my patients. Not only do you have to know what you are eating, but the crazy part about this is now you have to know what the animal ate, because what the animal ate can affect you. If the animal is given antibiotics, if the animal is given hormones, if the animal is eating omega-6, that is what you are getting.

There is one other one that people do not want me to talk about. This is a favorite: alcohol. I am not talking about moderate alcohol consumption for women, one glass of wine, three or four times a week or one drink three or four times a week, for guys, one glass a night, I am talking about excess alcohol consumption. It is rampant in our culture. I see couples come to me and they say, "Oh, every night my husband and I drink a whole bottle of wine, is that too much?" The answer is yes. High consumption of alcohol is linked to irritation and inflammation of the food pipe, the esophagus; we know that esophageal cancer is linked to alcohol consumption. Larynx, the voice box cancers, linked to alcohol consumption. And I know you find no surprise when I tell you that it affects the liver as well, everything from cirrhosis to alcohol-induced hepatitis and so on. So over time, chronic inflammation from alcohol can lead to tumor progression. You have to remember alcohol is a sugar. So if you are trying to keep your sugars down, you need to keep your alcohol down.

We will spend an entire lecture talking about sugar, and refined grains, white stuff, white bread, white rice, let me just leave it at this right now: Do not eat anything white. If it is white, find something else. Maybe with the exception of cauliflower; that one I want you to eat.

The last category we have is artificial food additives. This is the last one we need to look at as it relates to inflammation: things like monosodium glutamate, aspartame—these trigger the inflammatory response. So I think you know what I am getting at, do not buy anything in a package unless you can read the label, really clearly, and identify all of the ingredients. Again go back to whole food items, because you only find this stuff in packaged foods. One of the jokes I have with my patients is I say, "You can go to the supermarket, but walk around the outside aisles which basically puts them in the fruits and vegetable category. The minute you go into the middle of the supermarket where everything is packaged, you have to be like a detective."

Well, that is the bad news. There is a lot of stuff out there, and this stuff can really make us sick. So what do we do? How do we put out the fire? And how can we use food as medicine? So let's start with food first.

I have already talked to you about my whole foods, my love of whole foods, well, no surprise, what do I want you to eat to prevent inflammation? Whole grains, all the whole foods we have talked about, the fish high in omega-3, remember SMASH? Real kelp. That's right—seaweed. Kelp for example is very anti-inflammatory. But do not go buy it in a package where it is covered with all sorts of processed chemicals. You have to get it fresh. Again, whole fruits and vegetables, broccoli, blueberries, papaya, we talked about our shitake mushrooms. This is the first step. We also talked about oil, what oil do I want you to use? Of course, olive oil, avocado oil, macadamia nut oil, we are not going to be using corn oil, all of that leads to inflammation.

One category we did not hit on in previous lectures, is a category that is near and dear to my heart, which is tea. You may remember that in the nutrition lecture, not all foods are created equally. We talked about something called flavonoids. Flavonoids are phytonutrients. These phytonutrients have anti-inflammatory capacity. Now, tea is the second-most consumed beverage in the world next to water. So of course I want you to drink filtered water. Please do not drink your water from plastic bottles; it is not good for the environment, and as you will see in a later lecture, it is not good for you. Filtered water: That is number one. If you like tea, I want you to think about a few different teas. The first is black tea; beautiful research on black tea shows that black tea dilates blood vessels. You probably remember I once showed you a steak, and that steak constricted the blood vessel after you ate it. Well, black tea has the opposite effect. It dilates the blood vessel. Another favorite tea is green tea. Buy some organic green tea. Like broccoli, like turmeric, like shitake mushrooms, green tea can protect against cancer. It is anti-inflammatory, and as a matter of fact, a study came out of Japan showing that people who consumed just five little cups of green tea a day, five little ones, have a marked reduction in cardiovascular disease. So my two favorite drinks are tea and water.

One other tea worth mentioning is something called tulsi. Tulsi is an Ayurvedic herb; it comes from India. In India, tulsi is considered the herb of the deities. It is pure anti-inflammatory, and there are beautiful organic teas on the market where you can have green tea and tulsi together. To me, this is medicine.

We will spend a lot of time talking about herbs in a separate lecture. When I prepare food, I like to think about, what are the best kinds of spices, because spices, when used right, have powerful anti-inflammatory components. Now, I travel to India quite a bit, sometimes two times a year. And that is where I got introduced to turmeric. Because turmeric contains a powerful nontoxic compound called curcumin. Actually, this is what makes mustard have a yellow color. Research studies have shown that turmeric is as good, on occasion, as hydrocortisone and Motrin for inflammation. So think about that. Powerful drugs that are used to treat inflammation, we can get similar benefit from adding a spice. I like to add the turmeric to everything. You can add it to your kale; you can put it on top of your kale. I add it sometimes to egg whites—I like it there. You can put it anywhere that you want. In India they classically use it in the bean and lentil dishes. This is a common one. As you will see in the herbal medicine lecture, turmeric has anti-cancer properties. We even give our cancer patients turmeric two times a day to take.

The other great anti-inflammatory spice is ginger. Where might you think of using ginger? Well, you can put it in any food you like, if you like the taste of ginger, but as you will hear about in the herbal medicine lecture, we commonly use ginger for pregnant moms, we do not want to give a pregnant mom a pharmaceutical drug, if they have nausea, you can bet nine out of ten, or maybe ten out of ten holistic integrative physicians are going to recommend ginger. So ginger, like turmeric, has powerful anti-inflammatory benefits. It also has the added benefit of helping with nausea, with vomiting, not only related to cancer and chemotherapy, but also related to pregnancy.

Well, the list does not end there. There are a few more spices I like to use. You heard me mention tulsi. Well, you can remember that tulsi is also called holy basil. Basil in general, which is a staple in the Italian diet, is anti-inflammatory, as is rosemary. So if you like those, add them on. These are great spices that will decrease inflammation.

So we have been talking a lot about the causes of inflammation, and we now know not to eat sugar. We know which oils we should use, which oils we should put aside. We have some good food choices: whole foods, green vegetables, beans, and lentils. We know which spices we can use. I can tell you this: It works. I have seen it time and time again in my patients. We already talked about my corporate executive who came in with arthritis, skin rashes, said he needed a shot of steroids and antibiotics every month so he can go to his board meetings. And we took him off of gluten, which was causing his inflammation in the first place. He had food sensitivity.

But I had other patients have equally as miraculous cures. This was one of my favorites. I saw a veterinarian in his 50s who came to me because he was having a heart arrhythmia, something called atrial fibrillation. This is where the heart beats not regularly, jumps all around. And usually when we see this, we give blood thinners like Coumadin, and we give medications and today we have lots of surgical procedures, but he was not interested in any of that. So I said to him, "Tell me when your atrial fibrillation occurs?" and so he began to keep a journal, and he would have episodes maybe a minute, maybe 45 minutes, but invariably, they occurred when he ate sugar. So guess what? We had a simple treatment for his atrial fibrillation. I asked him to stop eating the sugar, and he said to me, "Why?" I said, "Because we have already identified it as a problem for you. But it is also inflammatory, and that inflammation is affecting your heart."

So at the end of the day, we have the power to put out the fire. If we just take these first steps I promise you, you will send me an e-mail, and you will say, "Dr. G., my arthritis is gone. Cleaned up my diet, got rid of the bad stuff, I no longer have pain." You will tell me that your energy is better; that you are sleeping better, and the list is endless. I remember when my corporate executive came back to the office. His head was down a little bit because he was giving me a hard time about stopping gluten. He did not really get it at first that the gluten was causing the inflammation, and the inflammation was causing the skin rashes and the arthritis. And he said to me, "I get it now, I finally realize that the health of my heart is in my hands."

Food Sensitivity and the Elimination Diet
Lecture 7

Illness can be connected to food in ways that you never thought about before. In this lecture, you will discover the six most common causes of food allergy and food sensitivity. You will learn how to eliminate these foods from your diet in a very scientific and practical way. You will also learn about some food options—such as drinking almond milk instead of cow's milk—that can lead to success with the elimination diet.

Food Allergies versus Sensitivities

- There are two types of reactions. An allergic reaction to a food happens quickly. It is a food allergy in which someone eats shellfish or a peanut, for example, and all of the sudden, they cannot breathe. The protein responsible for this is IGE.

- On the other hand, you may not recognize food sensitivity immediately. It is one of the causes of low-grade chronic inflammation. You keep taking in a food, and your body keeps seeing it as a foreign invader, and your body works constantly to clear the toxin from your system. Even though the reaction may not seem severe, the long-term consequences are enormous.

- Fatigue, trouble sleeping, mental fogginess, mood changes, irritability, anger, skin irritation, and rashes are common signs and symptoms of food sensitivity.

- Arthritis, muscle stiffness, and joint pain can be caused by the protein in cow's milk; it's not just about having gas and bloating. Nasal congestion, post-nasal drip, sinus infections, and ear infections can also be related to food sensitivity.

- If you have any of these signs and symptoms, there is a good chance that you have food sensitivity. More importantly, research has shown that the symptoms of food sensitivity are most likely connected to six common groups: dairy, gluten, corn, soy, peanuts, and egg.

The Elimination Diet

- The elimination diet is a dietary program that is designed to clear your body of foods that you may be allergic or sensitive to. For best results, you should stick with the diet—without exception—for two weeks. The tricky part is to not eat a group of foods either whole or as ingredients in other food; you must eliminate a group in its entirety.

- Start this program by eliminating all six common food irritants on day one. Before you start, you want to have a list of foods you can and cannot eat from your nutritionist, and you want to have the right foods in your house. Between days two and seven, you may start to feel like your symptoms are getting worse, but this is expected. As you clear your body of the toxins, sometimes they flare up. By about day eight, and somewhere between days eight and 14, your symptoms should disappear. If they do, then you know that one of those six food groups is causing your symptoms.

- To determine which of the six foods is causing your symptoms, on day 15, reintroduce one of those foods. Have a small amount for breakfast, some for lunch, and some for dinner. Then, stop consumption of that food after that day, and wait to see how your body reacts to the reintroduction of this food on days 16 and 17.

- You then continue cleaning everything out of your diet that you had eliminated over the course of two weeks by reintroducing them one at a time. Reintroduce a food, and wait for two days to monitor the response. Then, do not keep that food in your diet; keep it out until the elimination diet is over. This helps you identify which foods you are sensitive to. Many people are sensitive to more than one food.

- If you have sinus congestion, gas, and bloating in the abdomen, the target is usually dairy. The other big one is gluten. So, you can just eliminate those two most common allergens for two weeks as a shortcut to the process.

Substitutions for Common Allergens

- As a substitution for cow's milk, try drinking rice milk, coconut milk, or almond milk. However, try to stay away from soy milk because soy can be a very common food sensitivity item as well.

- The process of finding substitutions for nongluten grains is a little more complicated than substituting for milk. Two of the best substitutions are brown rice and quinoa. Others include buckwheat, arrowroot, and millet.

- You can buy gluten-free bread, such as bread made from organic brown rice, and you can use rice flour, quinoa flour, and potato flour for baking. However, because potato is white, it is not the healthiest option. You can even use garbanzo beans and rice bran as substitutions.

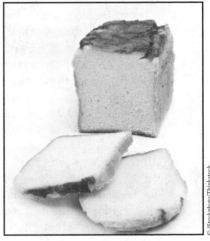

© iStockphoto/Thinkstock.

Gluten-free products, such as gluten-free bread, are readily available in many supermarkets.

- The other four items on the list of common allergens—corn, soy, eggs, and peanuts—are easier to avoid, but they are frequently hidden in various foods, so you should be aware of this and read food labels carefully.

- Be aware that baking powder frequently has cornstarch in it, and high fructose corn syrup comes from corn. In addition, the vinegar that is in condiments such as ketchup, mayonnaise, and mustard frequently comes from wheat or corn.

- Some breads are advertised as gluten-free, but they often contain oats, spelt, and rye. If you see the word "multigrain" on a product, it usually contains a mixture of things, and there is a good chance that it has gluten.

Tips for the Elimination Diet
- Make extra food at night so that you have some leftovers for the next day. If you are dedicating the time to cook and prepare healthy, anti-inflammatory foods when on the elimination diet, you should prepare extra.

- During this process, drink plenty of filtered water—but not water from plastic bottles. In addition, don't exercise too much during this time. Your body is clearing toxins, and it needs to heal. Do your best to walk outside every day for about 10 minutes, but don't do any heavy strength training or weight lifting, and don't engage in prolonged periods of exercise.

- When you start this diet, you may experience some fatigue, you may get a headache, and your joints may ache a little, but this is only because your body is withdrawing from these foods and cleansing your body of toxins.

- When you start craving the foods you have eliminated, stick with the program. These symptoms don't last long, so be strong.

- Get the guidance and support that you need. You have the ability to transform your life if you are able to eliminate allergens from your diet.

Questions to Consider

1. What are the top six food allergens?

2. What is the purpose of the elimination diet?

Food Sensitivity and the Elimination Diet
Lecture 7—Transcript

Welcome back. I always say that the greatest things I have learned have come from my patients. One weekend I went to a holistic integrative medicine conference and I heard about food sensitivity and food allergies. This is one of those areas that Western medicine does not teach very well. I never really learned about it in medical school. So I came back to work on Monday and as luck would have it, a young woman showed up in my office, and she said, "I do not really know why I am here. My mother forced me to come see you. I am getting married in two weeks and I have to have sinus surgery." So I thought this is going to be interesting. She said, "I do not want to have the sinus surgery because I do not want it to interfere with my wedding pictures." Why was she having sinus surgery? Well, for the last year, she had been on antibiotics six times, a course of 10 days each time. She was living on antibiotics because of her sinuses. I said to her, "You know what, I just heard some of the most amazing data as it relates to food and illness." I said, "If I take you off of the common food allergens, would you be willing to do it, and we can see if we can impact your sinuses." And she said to me, "Yes." So I did. About six months later she showed up in my office with a new last name, because now she was married. And I said to her, "How are you doing?" and she said to me, "I'm cured." The most important lesson that we can learn from this person, my patient, is illness can be connected to food in ways that we never even thought about.

Today's lecture will explore common food sensitivities, and one very successful strategy for dealing with them, the elimination diet.

Let's start with a few definitions. I mentioned in a previous lecture that there are two types of reactions; one is an allergic reaction that happens quickly. This is a food allergy in which someone eats shellfish, or they eat a peanut, and all of the sudden they can't breathe. The immune globulin, the protein responsible for this, is IGE. But food sensitivity is something different; you may not recognize it immediately. It is one of those causes of low-grade chronic inflammation, which we talked about. You keep taking in a food, and your body keeps seeing it as the enemy. It is that foreign invader. It is that toxin. And the body is working 24/7 to clear it from your system.

Even though the reaction may not seem severe, meaning you have trouble breathing, the long-term consequences are enormous.

What are some of the signs and symptoms that we expect to see with food sensitivity? I see these again every day. Fatigue, trouble sleeping, mental fogginess, people who say to me, "I can't focus, and I lose my concentration." We can even see mood changes—irritability, anger, these are very common. And if you have any of these, I want you to start writing them down. Think about what I am saying, because although this program may not be for everyone, if you have any of these symptoms or signs, this may be just what you need. Skin irritation, rashes, "Oh, I have eczema." "Oh I have psoriasis." All of these have been linked to food sensitivity. What about something as simple as arthritis? Joint pain? I mentioned in a previous lecture that the casein, the protein in milk, cow's milk, can cause arthritis. It is not just about gas and bloating. Muscle stiffness. You may have gas and bloating, you may have what we call Irritable Bowel Syndrome, diarrhea one day, constipation the next. Remember that patient that had the sinusitis? What did she have? She had nasal congestion, post-nasal drip, sinus infection, ear infections; she had all of those, and they were related to food sensitivity.

If you have any of these signs and symptoms, there is a good chance that you have food sensitivity. More importantly, research has shown that your symptoms are most likely connected to six common groups. These include: 1) diary; 2) gluten; 3) corn; 4) soy; 5) peanuts; 6) egg. These are the six common food sensitivity items that we see.

How do we determine if your symptoms are coming from one of these six foods? Well, there is a tried and true method; it is called the elimination diet.

The elimination diet is a dietary program, which is designed to clear your body of foods that you may be allergic or sensitive to. When we get into the protocol, we will ask you to stick with the diet without exception for two weeks. Now the tricky part to this is to not eat the foods whole or as ingredients in other food. What do I mean by that? Well, many people say to me, "Oh I can give up dairy; I do not drink much milk." And then I say, "Well, it is also in pizza cheese," and I see a sad face come on. Dairy is also whey, casein, lactose, so when we talk about eliminating a group, we eliminate it in its entirety. You may be thinking gee, I don't know if I can figure this all out. Well, there are certainly great websites to help you. And definitely eating out during this time can be a challenge. But what I do with my patients is I have them sit with a nutrition expert who really understands the elimination diet, and we are able to walk my patients right through with what to eat and what not to eat.

So how do we do this? Where do we begin? Well, let's say you are really suffering with arthritis. Or, you have really bad Irritable Bowel Syndrome. I want you to do this program right from the beginning by eliminating all six food irritants. So on day one, we begin the elimination diet. And before you start, of course you want to have from your nutritionist the foods you can and can't eat, just to help you out, and you want to have the right foods in your house, you want to be ready. Now, between day two and day seven, you may start to feel like your symptoms are getting worse. You may say, "Well, my arthritis is a little worse," or, "All of the sudden, my skin rash has come back out." This is what we expect. As you clear your body of the toxins, sometimes they flare up. In traditional Chinese medicine we call this a healing crisis; it is part of the healing. By about day eight, and somewhere between day eight and day 14, the symptoms should resolve. They should disappear. If they do, then we know we have hit a home run. One of these six food groups is causing your symptoms.

Now the big question is: Which food is it? I just gave up soy, I gave up dairy, I gave up gluten, I gave up corn, I gave up eggs, I gave up peanuts. I gave up all six; I feel great. But which one is it?

So, on day 15, we want you to reintroduce one of those foods, for example, dairy. Have some dairy in the morning, a small amount in the a.m. Have it again for lunch. And have a small amount for dinner. And then stop; stop the dairy after that day. And now we wait. We wait and see what our body does with reintroducing this food. So on day 16 and 17, we wait for the body's reaction. What do I expect to hear from my patients? Frequently at this time, people say, "Oh, I ate the ice cream and my sinusitis, my sinuses flared up. I knew right away it was ice cream; I knew it was dairy." So this is how we do it. By day 18, we are ready to re-introduce the second food. Let's say the second food is gluten, so now we reintroduce the gluten. And we do the same thing. Small amount in the morning, and a little bit more in the afternoon, and later in the day. And this process will go on until we get through all six food groups. So let's review: We clean everything out of the diet that we discussed for two weeks, we reintroduce them one at a time. We reintroduce a food, and we wait for two days to see the response. And then we do not keep that food in our diet, we keep it out until the elimination diet is over. This helps us to identify which foods we are sensitive to. And many of us are sensitive to more than one food.

I have to take a minute to share my own story. I am a milk baby. I love milk. I have loved it my entire life, as a kid and as an adult. I can drink a quart of milk a day. And I would always have organic fat-free milk. And I all of the sudden began to get arthritis. And I thought this is bizarre, my joints are hurting. So when I did the elimination diet, I found it was related to dairy. Stopping the dairy stopped the inflammation in my joints. I do not say I like it, but I really like not having joint pain, and I have substitutes for my dairy, which we will talk about later on. So again, remember, introduce one food for one day, and then do not reintroduce it back into your diet until you complete going through all six foods.

I bet some of you are saying, "This is too much, I do not think I can do this, seems too intense." Well, there is a little shortcut that I use with some of my patients, and I am going to tell it to you. If my patient says, "I always have flare-ups of my sinuses, I have post-nasal drip," like the lady I presented in the beginning. Already the bells are going off to me as a physician, "She's got a sensitivity to dairy." That is number one. So when I hear about sinus congestion and gas and bloating in the abdomen, I am usually targeting dairy. The other big one is gluten. And so if you can just do the two most common allergens, eliminate those two for two weeks. Dairy, including all milk, cream, cheese, cottage cheese, yogurt, butter, ice cream, frozen yogurt, you have to look where it is and it is added into a lot of things. The same with gluten. Wheat, spelt, oats, rye, barley, malt, you have to get the list and you have to take those out. Those two for many people solve the problem. But some people do have other food sensitivities as we mentioned.

Now that we have some of the basics, let's take a look at some of the research, because this may seem like it is not for real, it may seem like it is too simple, or it is impossible. But, there is strong evidence to support what I am saying. I like this study that appeared in *The Lancet* in 1979. It looked at people who were having migraine headaches on a routine basis. For those of you who have migraines, I want you to really think about the elimination diet, because what this study showed was that 78 percent of the people who suffered from migraines had a sensitivity to wheat. That is where the gluten comes in. Other sensitivities were also identified like egg, 45 percent; for some it was milk, 37 percent. And then there were a few others, some people were actually sensitive to oranges, to citrus, some to beef, corn even came up over 30 percent of the time. What sold me on this study was when you looked at the number of headaches that people had. On average for the whole group, they had 402 headaches per month. For those of you who have migraines, this is a crippling, crippling phenomenon. Those people who identified the foods they were sensitive to, who did the elimination diet; their headaches fell as a group from 402 to six per month. That is huge, 402 to six. In this study, 85 percent of the people became headache free. That, to me, is powerful medicine.

What about people who have Irritable Bowel Syndrome? This is common. "I have gas, I have bloating," we have talked about this. Well, they did a very similar study, and this appeared in *The Lancet*. Basically, what they did was place people on the elimination diet, and then looked for the foods that were the triggers for their symptoms. What they found was this: Number one was wheat, corn, and dairy. Again, we see those common culprits coming up, those common foreign invaders, if you might, that trigger the entire inflammatory response. Coming off the foods, resolution of symptoms.

Well, I know you think this may be a little complicated. And as I told my patient, and she had two weeks to get married, I said, "I am going to give you some quick substitutions that you can do right now to replace the common food sensitivity or food allergens." So, when I told her to come off of dairy, I said, "You have lots of options." Have rice milk. Have coconut milk. Have almond milk. I did not give her soymilk because remember, we said soy can be a very common food sensitivity item. She said, "I like rice milk," and that is what she drank.

A little bit more complicated than that is the non-gluten grains. But once we learn what they are, it really is pretty easy. I will just give you my two favorites: brown rice and quinoa. There are others, buckwheat, arrowroot, for example, millet, but most people feel pretty good just working with the brown rice and the quinoa. Now, you may notice, when you go to buy gluten-free products, and there are many today on the market, some are made with potato flour. That is not my favorite. My favorite ones are made with organic brown rice.

If you want to bake, if you want to make breads, what would you use? Well, you certainly can go and buy a gluten-free bread, like one made from organic brown rice. You can use rice flour for baking. You can use quinoa flour. You can use potato flour. But again, because remember, potato is white, it's not my favorite item. Amaranth. You can even use garbanzo bean, and that is a surprise. You can use arrowroot. You can use rice bran. So we have some good options. Again, for me, quinoa and organic brown rice being the favorites.

If you like a nice warm cereal in the morning like an oatmeal, well, you can get a gluten-free variation on that, and they are quite good. You can also have cream of rice if you like that. Instead of having wheat flakes, you can have puffed rice; you can have quinoa flakes. If you decide, "Gee, I want a bowl of pasta," well, it does not have to be wheat pasta, it can be rice pasta, for example. And I also like to get those little rice crackers, they have hardly any calories, they are made organically, you can eat 10 and you do not even get 100 calories, and they taste really good. So rice crackers are a good option.

Remember, when you are substituting for dairy, think about nuts, and think what kind of milk-type products can I get that come from the nut? And my favorite here is almond milk. But you can also get coconut milk, and you can get rice milk. All of these are readily available in any supermarket, easy to buy. Again, I like to buy them organic whenever possible—especially the almond milk.

The other four items on our list are easier to avoid. But, I have to mention that they are frequently hidden in things. If I tell you not to eat corn, you know not to eat corn. Soy is a little bit trickier, because there are large numbers of vegetarian meats, lots of them, on the market, that have soy in them. Soy is also in soy sauce, tofu, and miso. Soy is added to a lot of things, so again, you want to read your labels and you want to read them carefully.

Sometimes eggs are another added ingredient. So you have to look at the label. And peanuts. So corn, soy, eggs, and peanuts, those are the other four we want you to avoid.

I had something happen to me on Christmas Eve. I had a friend come to visit, and she is a chef, she has written a number of cookbooks. And I was thrilled to have her help cook; that was a good thing. I was not thinking; I let my guard down. She made a spinach dish. I love spinach. I ate a big portion of the spinach dish, and when my stomach began to act up, I realized, and I said to her, "Did you put cream in the spinach?" and she said "I made it with cream," and I thought, "No wonder I am having this problem." So remember, no creamed vegetables. And no corn added to the vegetable. So if you have a mixed vegetable, it can't have corn in it. Sometimes, we forget.

There are a few other pitfalls worth watching out for. If you tend to use baking powder, for example it frequently has cornstarch in it. All of those products that are on the market that say high fructose corn syrup, I do not want you to eat those anyway, I mean, I do not want you to eat anything that has high fructose corn syrup, but just remember, that is corn. And then one that I did not think about was vinegar. Because the vinegar that we have in condiments like ketchup and mayonnaise and mustard frequently comes from wheat or corn. So we have to be detectives, and again this goes back to working with a nutritionist. It is really helpful, here.

We need to read our food labels super carefully. Some breads are advertised as gluten-free, yet they contain oats and spelt and rye. You want to make sure, even if you were someone who ate tuna fish, for example, that it didn't have a soy filler in the tuna. This is common. If you see the word multi-grain on a product, it has usually got a mixture of things, so for example multigrain rice cakes. There is a good chance that they have gluten. Rice cakes are not my favorite food because they are white. But, for the two weeks of the elimination diet, if you need them for a snack, that is okay. I really prefer the pure rice crackers, myself.

Let's go through some tips. I always encourage my patients to [make] food at night so they have some leftovers for the next day. If you a[re] through the time to cook and prepare good anti-inflammatory food[s] certainly if you're doing the elimination diet, this is a great time to ha[ve] extra. You can also prepare extra. You can make a little bit extra chicken, for example, you can make a little bit extra sweet potato. You can make those foods that you enjoy and have them as leftovers.

Remember, your body is going to change with this elimination diet. The first few days, you might feel more symptoms, by day eight, you are going to feel much better. But during this process, we want you to drink plenty of filtered water. Remember, not water from plastic bottles. Good old fashioned plain filtered water. I also do not like you to exercise too much during this time. Your body is clearing toxins, it needs to heal. This is a healing program. So do your best to walk, get out in the sun every day for 10 minutes, but not too heavy strength training and weight lifting and prolonged periods of exercise. Do not add that burden to your body for just these two weeks.

What we have done today is to identify the six most common causes of food allergy and food sensitivity. We have learned how to eliminate them from our diet in a very scientific and practical way. We have discussed some food options, for example, almond milk instead of cow's milk. And these can really lead to success with the program.

It is true when you start this diet, you may experience a little bit of fatigue, you may get a headache, your joints may ache a little bit more. Remember what I said about healing crisis. Your body is withdrawing from these foods, and it is cleansing your body of toxins.

Your body might start saying to you, "Eat the gluten. Eat the dairy." When you start craving those foods, stick with the program. These symptoms don't last long. I need you to be really, really strong to do this. Get the guidance and the support that you need. I have seen people's lives transformed when they eliminate the allergens from their diet. I promise you this: You will tell me that the end result is absolutely 100 percent positively worth it.

Lecture 8

and supplements play an important role in our health.
...lecture, you are going to learn how to base your decision to
V take any natural product on good evidence and how to choose the best dietary supplements. There are supplements for the brain, heart, and gut. Most importantly, supplements are just supplements—they are not a replacement for proper nutrition and a healthy lifestyle. Before you start a supplement program, consult a physician.

Dietary Supplements

- Not everyone needs the same supplement. In addition, people do not need the same supplement all the time.

- We all need to be informed consumers when it comes to the natural products industry. Today, 52 percent of adults in the United States take some form of a dietary supplement, and 30 percent of U.S. children take dietary supplements on a regular basis. The natural products industry is a 23-billion-dollar industry.

The Regulation of Dietary Supplements

- In 1994, the Dietary Supplement Health and Education Act (DSHEA) was passed, ruling that products listed as dietary supplements are not required to undergo the same stringent approval as drugs. In addition, they do not require proof of safety and effectiveness.

- DSHEA also mandated that a supplement could not claim to diagnose, treat, cure, or prevent a disease, and every dietary supplement had to have a disclaimer on it stating that fact. Unfortunately, this did not stop people who wanted to make money, and products named BP Low, for example, appeared in the market with the assumption that it would lower your blood pressure—even if it couldn't.

- Even after DSHEA was passed, there were many supplements on the market that had prescription medications in them. For example, in 2002, a supplement called PC-SPES was found to have a blood thinner called Coumadin and an antianxiety drug called Xanax in it. Clearly, there needed to be further legislation and regulation.

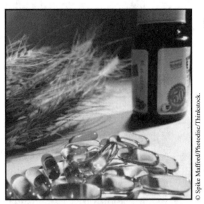

- In 2007, the good manufacturing practice (GMP) law was passed, requiring safeguards on manufacturing dietary supplements. It requires that dietary supplements are manufactured **In the medical community, there is a lot of controversy about whether dietary supplements can cure people's ailments.** consistently in terms of their identity (that what is in the bottle is what it says is in the bottle), purity (that it does not contain added heavy metals, sawdust, or prescription medications, for example), strength, and composition.

- Later in 2007, the U.S. FDA mandated that if a product has a problem, it needs to be reported to them within 15 days and that every supplement bottle has to have on its label information about who makes it and where the report should be sent. This has resulted in many supplements being recalled.

- There are some companies that do independent testing of GMP guidelines. For example, ConsumerLab.com does both voluntary and nonvoluntary testing of dietary supplements. They are an independent body that gives out a lot of free information and puts their seal of approval on a bottle once they test the supplement.

- The United States Pharmacopeia (USP) label, like the GMP label, implies that identity, strength, purity, and quality of the supplement has been evaluated. In other words, the product contains the ingredients it says it has.

- Another independent certification body is the National Science Foundation (NSF). They also certify the content in natural supplement bottles.

- Most importantly, when a supplement is tested by a reputable source, make sure that if you take that supplement, you are taking the one that was studied. If you take one that looks like it but is not the one that was tested, it may not give you the same result.

- In addition to ConsumerLab.com, you can get information about supplements on www.naturaldatabase.com and on the NIH's website.

The Benefits of Natural Products
- Probiotics are found in yogurt, kefir, and many other food items. A probiotic is a living organism that, when ingested in the right amounts, can have a healthy benefit on the host—a human being, in this case.

- Acidophilus is a common example of a probiotic. Lactobacillus is another one, and there are some patented probiotics that are on the market that are quite good.

- One of the most serious inflammatory diseases is ulcerative colitis, which can make someone's life miserable by causing dehydration, nausea, gas, bloating, and diarrhea. Probiotics improve flare-ups of ulcerative colitis.

- People who have gastroenteritis, or inflammation of the gastrointestinal (GI) tract, often experience diarrhea, which dehydrates them as a result of the loss of fluids. They lose potassium and magnesium, which is why they feel so terrible. If they take probiotics, there is a significant reduction in the risk and duration of diarrhea.

- Antibiotics, when taken on a routine basis, can change the entire bacteria of your bowel—the flora of your intestinal tract—so much that a pathogen begins to grow, causing profound diarrhea. Probiotics can prevent antibiotic-induced diarrhea and help with the symptoms.

- In addition, studies have shown that giving probiotics to people along with any antibiotics that they are taking has the potential to decrease morbidity, health-care costs, and mortality. This effect has been proven in children as well as adults.

- Selenium, another natural supplement, was studied in the 1990s. Participants in a study that was published in the *Journal of the American Medical Association* were given 200 mcg of selenium per day in hopes that it could protect against skin cancer. Although the selenium did not seem to have any effect on skin cancer, the study showed that prostate cancer decreased by over 50 percent and colorectal cancer decreased by over 60 percent.

- Vitamin D—which is not a vitamin, but is a hormone—is needed for your bones and heart. It protects your muscles, and it helps with depression and symptoms of fibromyalgia, such as muscle aching. Low levels of vitamin D can lead to calcification on the valves of the heart.

- A 2008 study showed that women with breast cancer who were deficient in vitamin D—with levels less than 50 ng/ml—had a 94 percent greater chance of metastatic disease and a 73 percent greater chance of death than patients with levels over 50 ng/ml.

- Taking four grams of omega-3 fish oil will lower your triglycerides—which is the form of fat that comes from sugar and white foods—by 45 percent.

- Niacin is a B vitamin that is used to correct a very important cholesterol abnormality. It raises the good cholesterol, or HDL.

Questions to Consider

1. What is DSHEA?

2. What does GMP mean?

Vitamins and Supplements
Lecture 8—Transcript

Welcome back. Today we get to talk about one of my favorite topics. Why is it a favorite? Because it is an area of a lot of controversy. It's all about natural supplements, natural products, vitamins, herbs, and other supplements.

Some people think that a supplement can cure everything, from hair growth to toenail fungus. I have colleagues that I work with on a daily basis that say, "Supplements are totally useless." Those are the two extremes.

Personally, I take a middle of the road approach. First I look at what my patients are eating, I do some blood work to see what they need, and then I make a decision on should I prescribe a supplement. So, let me give you a few examples. One of my favorite vitamins is vitamin D. Why might I use it? Well, if the vitamin D level is low, this can lead to depression, it can lead to symptoms of fibromyalgia, like muscle aching, it can lead to calcification on the valves of the heart. This is just a short list. Vitamin D isn't even a vitamin—it's a hormone. So that is one that I will measure the level of what is called the 25-hydroxy vitamin D, and I will give that to my patient. I may also use a B vitamin called niacin. Niacin is a tried and true B vitamin for correcting a very important cholesterol abnormality. Niacin raises the good cholesterol, the HDL. So I use niacin all the time in my practice, and we will also talk about some of the benefits of fish oil. These are just a few that I use every day.

As a physician, I have reached the conclusion that vitamins, herbs, and supplements do play an important role in our health. Today we are going to learn how to base your decision to take any natural product on good evidence, and how to choose the best ones.

I always smile when people show up in my office and they have a big bag of vitamins. Everything is in there, and I say, "Who advised you to take these?" and they say, "Well, my friend was telling me at the bridge club to take this or to take that." But, at the end of the day, not everyone needs the same supplement. For example, someone who has osteoporosis, well you can bet they are going to need things like calcium and vitamin D and K2, maybe even strontium, and zinc and magnesium to build their bones back. But that doesn't mean that everyone needs those things. We do not need the same thing all the time. For example, I mentioned the healing power of ginger. Well, if someone's going to take ginger in the form of a supplement, I usually give it for a particular reason, like if they are pregnant and they have nausea—that's a good time to give someone ginger in the form of a ginger tea, for example.

Most importantly we all need to understand the natural products industry. If we just go and pick things off the shelf, we are not making informed decisions; we need to make informed choices. To give you an idea of how important this is to be an informed consumer, let's take a look at some statistics.

We know today that 52 percent of adults in the United States take some form of a dietary supplement. This could be fish oil, it could be a B vitamin, it could be an antioxidant. Over 50 percent of the adult population. What was surprising to me in the research was that 30 percent of U.S. children take dietary supplements on a regular basis. And everyone is familiar with those little chewable vitamins that are given to kids. But 30 percent seemed like a big number. So what we are talking about here is a 23 billion dollar industry. This is big money. A lot of money is being spent, so clearly, there is a need for good information and education. So, let's take the first step and review how the dietary supplement industry is regulated. And, by the way, if you are thinking it is totally unregulated, there is no control, hopefully I am going to convince you that it is indeed regulated.

Well, we have to begin in the 1990s. In 1994, the Dietary Supplement Health and Education Act was passed. The acronym for this is DSHEA. So what did DSHEA say? DSHEA said that products listed as dietary supplements are not required to undergo the same stringent approval as drugs. Well that sounds scary. Also, they do not require proof of safety and effectiveness. So, basically, what that means is I can go in the back room here at The Great Courses, whip up a product, we can put a fancy label on it, and we can put it out as a dietary supplement in the '90s. I don't have to prove it is safe; I don't even have to prove it works. That is a scary piece.

What DSHEA also said was that you can't make a claim that you can diagnose, treat, cure, or prevent a disease with that supplement. So, for example, you could not say, "This supplement will lower your blood pressure." You could not say that. But that lead to bringing products on the market with names like BP Low. What does that imply to a person looking at the shelf? BP Low sounds like low blood pressure to me. Those kinds of things people were able to get away with. Every dietary supplement had to have a disclaimer on it. It had to say, "This statement has not been evaluated by the Food and Drug Administration. This product is not intended to diagnose, treat, cure, or prevent a disease." Well the sad part about this is this did not stop people who wanted to make money, and we saw products on the market like Cancer Off. Well that sounds like an anti-cancer thing to me. Cancer Off 126, and I would like to read the label to you because it is so amazing that this can exist. The label says, "This formula can help remove melanoma, breast cancer, lung cancer, intestinal cancer, lymphadenitis—that's inflammation of the lymph nodes—syphilis-related skin lesions." My God, this thing can cure everything. Just look at that. This is what gives natural supplements their bad reputation. This is bad medicine.

We also found, even after DSHEA, that there were many supplements on the market that had prescription medications in them. In 2002 for example, a supplement called PC-SPES, was found to have a blood thinner called Coumadin, and (amazing to me) Xanax (alprazolam), a drug that is like Valium. People were putting the drugs in the supplements. There were even supplements that were found to have sawdust in them. Products that said they could treat erectile dysfunction. In 2008 when they were analyzed found they had things like Viagra. So clearly, there is room for further legislation, and further regulation, and the good news is, it is happening.

In 2007 the good manufacturing practice law was passed. This requires safeguards on manufacturing dietary supplements. It requires that dietary supplements are manufactured consistently in terms of their identity, that what is in the bottle is what it says is in the bottle, its purity, it does not have added heavy metals, it does not have sawdust, it does not have prescription medications, its strength has to be verified, its composition, what it is made up of. So the good manufacturing practice has been required of natural supplement companies. Just a few months later in December of 2007, the

FDA said, "If a product has a problem, it needs to be reported to the FDA within 15 days. Mandatory reporting. And every supplement bottle has to have on the label information about who is making it, and where the report should go to." This has resulted in many supplements being recalled. The PC-SPES, which I talked about having the Coumadin in it or the warfarin, was taken off the market. Cancer Off, taken off the market. And you might think, "Gee, I am smart enough, I know not to buy those things, I know better, I am an educated consumer." But think about someone with cancer. They are looking for hope. They are looking for a cure, anything that can help them. And this becomes a million dollar industry leading to billions of dollars at the end of the day.

I have some other good news. Along with our GMP practices, there are some companies that are doing independent testing on their own. And there is a website I just want to call your attention to. The website is www. consumerlab.com. Consumer Lab does both voluntary, meaning I give them my supplement to test, and non-voluntary testing of dietary supplements. So that means they will actually go into the stores, take the bottles off the shelf, and test them. And what they are looking for is what we just talked about. They want to know: Does the supplement have the amount of strength, composition, identity, and purity that it says on the label?

So they are an independent body that gives out a lot of free information, to even people like me. When I am looking for the best product for my patients, for example, I went on consumerlab.com not too long ago, because I wanted to see what they rated as the best red yeast rice. That is a common supplement used to lower cholesterol. So I went on to consumerlab.com, took a look at what they were rating, and I was able to find the one that had the highest rating.

They also put their seal of approval on the bottle. It looks like an Erlenmeyer flask, one of those flasks you get in your chemistry class. And the flask will say, "CL"—Consumer Lab—tested. So if you see that, you at least know this product has been put through a series of tests, and it has passed in terms of its purity and its composition.

So watch out for the labels on the bottles. Look for the CL, look for the GMP—good manufacturing practice—and look for one more: USP. The USP label, like the GMP label, implies that identity, strength, purity, and quality of this supplement has been evaluated. These products that the ingredients they say they have. USP stands for United States Pharmacopeia.

So these products are made to what we call pharmaceutical grade. That means they are as good a product as if it was a drug, in terms of how it is made.

Another independent certification body is the NSF. They also certify the content in the natural supplement bottle. So again, if you see the CL for Consumer Lab, the GMP, the USP, or the NSF labels, you can feel relatively comfortable that this is a tested product. And, if you like to go to the Internet, I can give you lots of other resources.

Every year at Scripps, I do a conference on natural supplements, and I have to teach this to physicians. One of the resources I use for them is naturaldatabase.com. So you can go to www.naturaldatabase.com, and you can get information on supplements, on supplement drug interactions, anything you want to know. The second one I use quite a bit, again with physicians, is the dietary-supplements.info.nih.gov. This is the NIH's website. This is the NIH office of natural supplements. You can start with these two, and consumerlab.com, and you have three powerful websites that can help you immediately to navigate this industry.

The FDA also has a website for reporting adverse events. So if you think you have taken a product that has caused a problem for you, you can go to the fda.gov/medwatch website. Or, you can even call; they have a 1-800 number (1-800-FDA-1088). So lots of resources are now available to regulate an industry that for many years was not doing a great job. This industry is regulated.

So now we have some idea of how we can objectively evaluate natural products, vitamins, minerals, supplements, herbs, and we will have a whole lecture on herbal medicine alone. We know that there is a time and place for vitamins and supplements. But I just want to share with you a few that are on the market today that I want you to think about. And for the rest of the course, we will be talking about natural products throughout.

Let's start with one that is familiar to most people. It is called a probiotic. Now, you see probiotics showing up everywhere. They are in yogurt, they are in kefir, they are in lots of food items now. What is a probiotic? A probiotic is a living organism. It is a live organism that, when ingested in the right amounts, can have a healthy benefit on the host. The host would be us. So think about this for a second. That patient of mine, who I talked about with sinusitis in a previous lecture, took six courses of antibiotics, 10 days or so each, over the previous year. She was getting a lot of antibiotics. We know that when you take antibiotics, they do not just kill, if you might, the bad bacteria, they change the entire bacteria of your gut, the flora of your intestinal tract. This is one of the key reasons that people end up with gas and bloating after taking antibiotics. They do not have the healthy bacteria, it has been wiped out, and it has been replaced with unhealthy bacteria. So what are some examples of a probiotic? Acidophilus, that's a common one. Lactobacillus is another one. And there are some patented probiotics that are on the market that are quite good, for example, VSL#3 has eight different strains of probiotic. So let's take a look at some of the research on probiotics.

One of the most serious inflammatory diseases that we see is ulcerative colitis. Ulcerative colitis can not only make someone's life miserable, with some people having 100 bowel movements a day—and that is not an exaggeration at all, it is real, it is not exaggerated—they feel dehydrated, nauseous, gas, bloating, diarrhea. This is a tough disease to have.

They did a very interesting study. They said, "What if we take people with active ulcerative colitis, and we give them six grams a day of VSL#3." Remember, I said that is the probiotic that has eight different strains of the good bacteria (the lactobacillus, the acidophilus), eight different types of strains. They found that 85 percent of the people taking the VSL#3 were in remission one year later, versus only six percent of the placebo group. So to me, this is powerful medicine. Anyone with active ulcerative colitis needs to talk to their physician about being on probiotics. What is important here, I was very careful to tell you which product, because the product is the key. When a supplement is tested, you want to make sure if you take that supplement, you are taking the one that was studied. If you take one that looks like it, it may not give you the same result. An 85 percent reduction in symptoms still in remission, no symptoms versus six percent in placebo, that is unbelievable, from a probiotic.

Let's look at another indication for probiotics: people who have gastroenteritis—there is that -itis word again—inflammation of the GI tract. Maybe you got exposed to a bug like the rotavirus. Many children get exposed to a virus called rotavirus. And it can cause diarrhea. When you have a lot of fluid loss through your bowels, like diarrhea, you are going to get dehydrated. You are going to lose your potassium, lose your magnesium. That is why people feel so terrible—they are completely dehydrated. And what they found was that if you just give probiotics, you have a significant reduction in the risk of the diarrhea. That is huge. And you can correct the diarrhea associated with the rotavirus, meaning if someone has this acute virus, and you give the probiotics, you can slow down its course. And that is profound.

One other indication, and I sort of alluded to this earlier: A beautiful study came out that said, what if we give some good probiotics like lactobacillus—and the names right now are not so important because the research is there—what if we get people to consume 100 grams in the form of a drink of lactobacillus and other probiotics, and we have them do this two times a day while they are getting antibiotics, and for one week after their antibiotic course? Can we reduce the risk of antibiotic-induced diarrhea?

Now, I have to step back a bit. Antibiotics, when taken on a routine basis, and for some people even one course can change the bowel flora so much that *C. difficile* which is a pathogen begins to grow. *C. difficile* will cause the most profound diarrhea anyone ever can have, leading to all the problems I just discussed. What they found in this study, which was published in the *British Medical Journal*, was that those people taking the probiotic had a reduction of 21.6 percent of getting *C. difficile*. What they concluded was this: This has the potential to decrease morbidity, health care costs, and mortality if we just give the probiotics to people with their antibiotics. And this has been proven in children, as well.

So at the end of the day, we can conclude that probiotics improve flare-ups of ulcerative colitis. Remember, 85 percent of patients remained in remission, 85 percent. Prevent antibiotic-induced diarrhea, and help with the symptoms and shorten the duration of the diarrhea that is caused by gastroenteritis viruses like the rotavirus.

Well, what else is out there? Let's take a look at a few more. Let's look at selenium. Selenium was studied in the 1990s, and someone thought that maybe selenium could protect against skin cancer. So, they gave people participating in the study 200 mcg per day of selenium. Well, the endpoint of this study was skin cancer, and the selenium did not seem to have any effect. So, many people said, "Well you do not need the selenium." But what did the study show? The study showed that prostate cancer decreased by over 50 percent, and colorectal cancer by 62 percent. And this was in *The Journal of the American Medical Association*. Just giving selenium, 200 mcg per day. And that is a natural supplement.

Let's go back to vitamin D. You heard me say in the beginning vitamin D is needed for your bones, it is needed for your heart, it protects your muscles, it helps with symptoms of fibromyalgia, it helps with depression, it does all of these things. What about cancer? Is there any role for vitamin D in cancer? Well, a very interesting study was presented in 2008 at the American Society for Clinical Oncology. Basically, they know that breast cancer cells have vitamin D receptors. So they said, "Let's take a look at the vitamin D levels of the women with breast cancer." What they found is that 37 percent of the women had levels less than 50 nanograms/milliliter, 38 percent had levels between 50 and 72 nanograms/milliliter, and these are standard units. And, only 24 percent of the women had vitamin D levels that were greater than 72 nanograms/milliliter. This was not an overnight study. They followed 512 women for 11.6 years. And this is what they concluded: Those patients who were deficient in vitamin D, that was a level less than 50 nanograms/milliliter, 94 percent greater chance of metastatic disease, and a 73 percent greater chance of death than patients with levels over 50 nanograms/milliliter. So when a woman comes to see me, I say, "We are getting a vitamin D level on you, 25-hydroxy vitamin D." And when people say to me, "What level do you supplement to?" I usually say, "To around 55 nanograms/milliliter, based on this data."

I will be spending a lot of time in the natural treatments of cholesterol talking about supplements, because that is where I really use them a lot in my practice. But I would like to mention omega-3 fish oil. Taking fish oil four grams a day will lower your triglycerides 45 percent. That is the form of fat that comes from sugar, from cookies, cakes, candy and ice cream, white foods, white rice, and white bread, which hopefully no one after these lectures is eating.

This sample of studies, to me, clearly confirms that vitamins and supplements have an important, crucial impact on our health. They can't be ignored. We can't just simply say, "Don't take any vitamins or supplements." But it is important to remember that if you go out, and you choose a supplement based on some of the research that you use the same supplement that was in the study, that you use the same dose, even the same company, that way it has all the same manufacturing characteristics. Do not go and say, "Dr. G. said take probiotics if you have active ulcerative colitis," and go and pick some strange probiotic off the shelf. Go and get the one that works. And of course, before you start a supplement program, you need to speak to your physician. And, if you can't have the conversation with your physician, find one that you can talk to.

Remember: As you will hear throughout this course, there are supplements for the brain, supplements for the heart, and as you already heard, supplements for the gut. Most importantly, supplements are just that, they are a supplement; they are not a replacement for proper nutrition and a healthy lifestyle.

Herbal Remedies
Lecture 9

In this lecture, you are going to learn about herbal remedies. You will explore some of the ailments that they are used for and the evidence to support their use. Most pharmaceutical drugs come from botanicals, so herbal medicine is not alternative medicine. Herbs are powerful medicine, and when used in the correct formulations and doses, they can have a profound effect on health—from treating common, everyday ailments to more challenging chronic diseases.

Gastrointestinal Herbs

- Aloe vera is used to treat burns and wounds externally, but when taken internally, aloe vera is also used to treat the inflammation associated with mouth ulcers, mucositis—an inflammation of the lining of the mouth—from chemotherapy, and any irritation in the gastrointestinal tract, including colitis.

- The powdered aloe vera leaf is a potent laxative that works well to treat constipation. Because it is a strong laxative, use it with caution.

- Ginger is used to treat nausea and vomiting from pregnancy and chemotherapy or from any nausea in general. Ginger is the most extensively studied herb for nausea and vomiting.

- A review of over six clinical trials found that 1.5 grams per day of ginger is effective for treating pregnancy-induced nausea and vomiting. More importantly, research shows that ginger is safe—that there are no side effects or adverse events.

- A National Cancer Institute–funded study showed a 40 percent reduction in chemotherapy-induced nausea when people were given one half to one gram of ginger three days prior to chemotherapy and for the following week.

- Today, 25 million Americans suffer from heartburn, and one of the best herbal remedies for heartburn is licorice.

- Before you decide to take licorice for your heartburn, stop eating heartburn-causing foods, such as cooked tomato sauce, excess caffeine, chocolate, carbonated beverages, fried foods, alcohol, foods that are very high in fat, and full-fat dairy products. You should also ask your physician to test you for a bacteria that causes heartburn called *Helicobacter pylori.*

- Licorice raises blood pressure and lowers potassium, but the form of licorice that you should take for heartburn is labeled "DGL," which is the form of licorice that does not raise your blood pressure. Take 600 to 800 milligrams about 20 minutes before your meal for up to six weeks or when needed.

- Peppermint is an herbal remedy for irritable bowel syndrome (IBS), which is a very common disorder that affects the large intestine. Cramping, pain, bloating, gas, diarrhea, and constipation are all signs of irritable bowel syndrome.

- Peppermint slows down the gastrointestinal tract. It slows down the movement of food from the oral cavity down to the colon and inhibits smooth muscle cell contraction. If the colon is not contracting or spasming, you have less pain.

- Make sure to buy peppermint as enteric coated tablets because if you take peppermint that's not enteric coated, it will cause heartburn.

Urogenital Herbs

- Cranberry is a natural antibiotic that helps to prevent bacteria from adhering to the lining of the bladder wall.

- In 2009, a study was published that focused on whether cranberries could reduce the frequency of recurrent urinary tract infections in women. The researchers found that women who drank four ounces of cranberry juice two times per day or took tablets of cranberry extract in the amount of 400 to 800 milligrams per day had a reduction in their urinary tract infections.

- A common problem that men have is waking up at night—sometimes three, four, or five times per night—to urinate. Another symptom that men complain about is that their urinary stream is slow or sluggish—not forceful. These are signs of prostate enlargement, or prostate hypertrophy.

- The most studied herbal remedy for prostate enlargement is saw palmetto, which can be taken two times per day in 160-milligram doses. Research has shown that saw palmetto significantly improves symptoms in people who have mild to moderate enlargement of their prostate gland, which means that they get up to urinate less frequently at night and their urinary stream is stronger.

Herbs and Migraines

- Butterbur is a traditional European herb that has been used for years to treat allergies, but more recently, butterbur has been shown to significantly decrease the amount of migraine headaches.

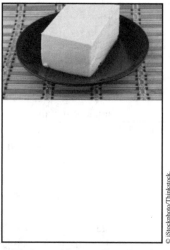

Butterbur, which can be taken for migraine headaches, is a plant that has broad leaves and purple flowers.

© iStockphoto/Thinkstock.

- In a placebo-controlled study, people who were given 150 milligrams of butterbur over a four-month period had a statistically significant reduction in their migraine headaches in comparison to a placebo group.

- Butterbur can have liver toxicity, which is why it's very important that, if it is the right herbal remedy for you, that you only use the herbal remedy that was studied—called Petadolex.

- Across 16 randomized controlled trials, butterbur did as well as prescription medications in reducing the number of migraine headaches.

- Studies have shown a 42 percent reduction in headaches in people taking just 300 to 400 milligrams of magnesium per day. Magnesium softens the stool if you are constipated, but if the stool becomes too soft, you have to cut back on it.

- In addition to butterbur in the form of Petadolex and magnesium, taking 400 milligrams per day of the B vitamin riboflavin can help reduce headaches.

- Omega-3 fish oil is anti-inflammatory, so you can take two to four grams per day. In addition, taking 300 milligrams per day CoQ10 has been shown to statistically reduce migraine headaches.

- Taking magnesium, omega-3 fish oil, and a low dose of riboflavin are the safest migraine-reducing choices if you are trying to become pregnant or are pregnant.

Herb-Drug Interactions
- Saint-John's-wort helps mild to moderate depression. However, if you're taking a medication—such as a birth control pill, heart medicine, or blood thinner—Saint-John's-wort can decrease the potency of the medication. Other medications will increase in their potency. Alcohol is amplified in the body when Saint-John's-wort is taken.

- The following four categories of prescription medications are the most common pharmaceutical drugs that have herb-drug interactions: blood thinners, sedatives, antidepressants, and diabetes medicine. If you are taking any type of medication within these categories, consult your physician before starting any natural remedies.

Questions to Consider

1. Which herbal remedy should be considered for irritable bowel syndrome?

2. Are all aloe vera preparations equivalent?

Herbal Remedies
Lecture 9—Transcript

Welcome back. Did you know that the bark of this tree is one of the most prescribed medications for headache and inflammation? Did you know that this beautiful flower has been prescribed by physicians for decades to treat heart arrhythmia? Well it's true. The first is white willow and I bet some of you take it every day. The bark of the white willow tree gives us aspirin and that beautiful flower is foxglove, which gives us an important heart medicine called Digoxin.

Let's stop thinking about herbs as alternative medicine. We have just seen that white willow and foxglove are used by physicians every day to treat common medical problems. Today, we are going to talk about a few of my favorite herbal remedies. We'll explore some of the ailments that they are good for and more importantly the evidence to support their use.

Let's start with four herbs that are great for the gastrointestinal tract. The first one in this category is aloe vera. Now you may think aloe vera is used to treat burns and wounds externally and you would be right. If I got a sunburn today, I would go in the garden, take some aloe vera from the plant, crack the plant open, and put that cool gel on my skin and it would definitely help the burn to heal. But, did you know that aloe vera is also used internally as well? Well I didn't know about that use of aloe vera internally. I actually learned it from a patient.

I remember when I was a young resident at Sloan-Kettering; we were treating a wonderful rabbi who had lymphoma. The chemotherapy was causing severe mouth ulcers; this is very common with chemotherapy. The rabbi came in one day and insisted that all of his mouth irritation and all of the ulcers were being relieved with the aloe vera. This was in the 1980s. Well guess what? The rabbi was right. Research has since shown that aloe vera, when taken internally, is indeed a soothing tonic for ulcers in the mouth, for sores, and for what's called mucositis. Mucositis is an inflammation of the lining of the mouth. And also internally aloe vera has been shown to help with the inflammation that we see in ulcerative colitis (an irritation to the colon lining).

Now, it's very important, as it is in all herbal medicine, to know what kind of formulations of herbal remedies that you are going to use. For example, for mouth ulcers you want to use the inner filet of the aloe leaf, two to three ounces two times per day. Why is it important to use the right one? Well aloe has a very special second indication. The powdered aloe vera leaf is a strong laxative. When I have patients who have really bad constipation I may recommend aloe vera and of course because it's a strong laxative we need to use it with a lot of caution.

Let's take a look at a second gastrointestinal herbal superstar. This one is ginger. Whenever I hear that someone has nausea, the first herb I reach for is ginger. Thirty to 55 percent of pregnant women will experience nausea and vomiting during their pregnancy; this is usually normal. Somewhere between week four and eight we see a lot of nausea and vomiting and then by week 16 a woman will say I feel great, all those symptoms are gone.

Ginger is the most extensively studied herb for nausea and for vomiting even in pregnant women. A review of over six clinical trials found that ginger, 1.5 grams a day is effective for treating pregnancy induced nausea and vomiting. What's even more important to me as a physician, the research shows that the ginger is safe, that there are no side effects or adverse events. It is not surprising that a National Cancer Institute funded study showed a 40 percent reduction in chemotherapy induced nausea when people were given ginger, one-half to one gram three days prior to chemotherapy and for the following week. Again, when I hear that someone has nausea, even if they're pregnant, especially if they're on chemotherapy I encourage them to use dried ginger.

Now, we have already seen two really good uses for herbal medicine. Number one, aloe vera to treat the inflammation associated with mouth ulcers, mucositis from chemotherapy, or any irritation in the GI tract, including colitis. Remember the powdered aloe vera can be a very potent laxative and works really well to treat constipation. Number two, ginger for nausea and vomiting from pregnancy, from chemotherapy, or just any nausea in general.

As a cardiologist, I see people who take many medications. One of the common ones is antacids. And patients ask me all the time Dr. G. can I get off the antacid? Well we know today that 25 million Americans suffer from what we call heartburn. Many of my patients want to put aside the prescription medications and they say give me something natural for my heartburn and one of my favorite herbal remedies in this situation to treat heartburn is licorice. But, I want you to do two things before you decide to take licorice for your heartburn. Remember food first; so number one, stop heartburn causing foods. Let's review what they are.

Cooked tomato sauce; this is a big one, very acidic. Excess caffeine, especially coffee, so don't be drinking seven cups of coffee a day and come in and tell me you have heartburn. Chocolate, soda, and any carbonated beverage, even carbonated water can cause heartburn. Some of the more obvious ones, fried foods, alcohol, foods very high in fat, your beef, your pork, and your lamb, and full fat dairy. So, food first. Clean out the diet.

Number two, before you look for a supplement for your heartburn, if this is a problem for you quite a bit, I want you to go to your physician and I want you to ask them to test you for a bacteria that causes heartburn called helicobacter pylori. Remember we talked about this bacteria as a cause of chronic inflammation and after you do those two, change your diet and check your blood for helicobacter pylori, then you can think about taking licorice.

There is one important thing you need to know about licorice. Licorice raises blood pressure, but the form of licorice that I want you to take will be labeled this way, DGL. This is the form of licorice that does not raise your blood pressure. So, if you suffer from heartburn routinely go and buy the licorice with the DGL on the label and take 600 to 800 milligrams about 20 minutes before your meal. Now I tried this, it tastes pretty good so you just chew on it 20 minutes before your meal and you can do this for up to six weeks or you may just want to take it when needed, at which point you can take anywhere from 300 to 400 milligrams as needed. Remember other forms of licorice can increase blood pressure and lower your potassium. A lot of people don't realize a common cause of high blood pressure is—guess what?—black licorice. Sometimes we just have patients stop their black licorice and even their black jelly beans and their blood pressure goes down.

The last superstar we will talk about for the GI tract is peppermint. Peppermint is a tried and true herbal remedy for irritable bowel syndrome. Now I have mentioned irritable bowel syndrome before. This is a very common disorder which affects the colon, the intestine, the large colon. Frequently people will say they cramping, pain, bloating, gas, diarrhea, and even constipation; these are all signs of irritable bowel syndrome. We already talked about the elimination diet and how it can help irritable bowel syndrome, but if you needed a supplement or an herbal remedy, peppermint is the way to go.

Research has shown two mechanisms for how peppermint works. The main one is peppermint slows down the GI tract. It slows down the movement of food from the oral cavity all the way down to the colon and it inhibits smooth muscle cell contraction. Think about this; if the colon is not contracting and it's not spasming, you have less pain. This helps the pain and the bloating that we frequently see with irritable bowel syndrome. An important caveat about peppermint, make sure you buy your peppermint as enteric coated tablets three times a day because if you take peppermint that's not enteric coated it will cause heartburn.

Well now we've evaluated some herbs for the gastrointestinal tract, let's take a look at some for the urogenital tract. Let's pick a problem women frequently face and one that men frequently face, urinary tract infections and prostate enlargement. In 2009, a study was published that looked at cranberry and the focus of the study was whether or not cranberry would reduce the frequency of recurrent urinary tract infections in women. What they found was that those women who drank four ounces two times a day of cranberry or took extracts, tablets of cranberry, 400 to 800 milligrams daily had a reduction in their urinary tract infections.

You may remember when we talked about the healing properties of food that I mentioned the cranberry actually is a natural antibiotic and it helps to prevent the bacteria from adhering to the lining of the bladder wall. If you suffer from recurrent urinary tract infections, you may want to try cranberry, four ounces two times a day if you like the juice, but please make it unsweetened. I don't want you to get the extra sugar and especially if you're diabetic, use the cranberry extract 400 to 800 milligrams per day.

What about for the guys? A common problem men come into my office with is waking up at night to urinate. Some men wake up three, four, or five times a night. Needless to say that doesn't make for a good night's sleep. The minute I hear that the first thing I'm thinking is how big is his prostate? A second symptom men complain about is that their urinary stream is slow or sluggish, not forceful. These are signs of what we call prostate enlargement or prostate hypertrophy.

What might we do in this situation? Well, the most studied herbal for prostate enlargement is saw palmetto. Research has shown that saw palmetto significantly improves the symptoms I just described in people who have mild to moderate enlargement of their prostate gland. That means they get up less frequently at night and their urinary stream is stronger. Saw palmetto has not been shown to make big improvements in people with severe, severe prostate symptoms, but in mild to moderate prostate enlargement it is as good as the pharmaceutical called Proscar. In fact, Proscar has the active ingredients of the botanical saw palmetto. If you decide you want to try saw palmetto you need to look at the label of the bottle; 160 milligrams two times a day. Remember if you're not certain if you have the right product, check the Consumerlab.com website as we discussed in our previous lecture because not all products are made the same.

How does this work in real practice? What happens when someone comes into my office with a medical problem and they say, "Dr. G., I want to go on supplements." How might I approach this person? What kind of questions would I ask before just putting someone on a supplement regimen?

Let's take a real person. Sally came to see me because she had a history of migraine headaches. She's 36 years old. She told me that she has a family history of migraine headaches as well, but she has suffered from migraines since she was age 14. Sally told me that her headaches occur four to 10 times per month and when they occur they are debilitating. She has to go to bed and take multiple medications. She's noticed some triggers for her migraines. She says they're worse when she drinks red wine, when she eats cheese, and around the time of her menstrual cycle. By the time she came to see me, she had seen many physicians. She was on the best that western medicine has to offer. She had the best drugs available to her. Her laboratory tests looked pretty good, nothing was abnormal, and she even had a brain MRI which was normal. They could not find a reason for her migraine headaches.

I say to Sally let's start with food first. Obviously we want to remove the triggers for your migraines. She'd already identified red wine and cheese, but given the number of headaches that Sally had I would probably have her do an elimination diet because as we have seen in a previous lecture the elimination diet can really impact migraine headaches. At a minimum, Sally needs to be on an anti inflammatory diet. We always go with the food first, whole foods, off of the carbohydrates, off the white stuff, the foods high in sugar and hopefully in Sally's case I can convince her to try the elimination diet. When I saw Sally, she was really eager to have a supplement.

So, I have to think about the research on all of the supplements as they relate to inflammation and in this case specifically as they relate to migraine headache. One of the first supplements I picked for Sally is called butterbur. Now, butterbur has been around for a long time. It's your traditional European herb that has been used for years for allergies, but more recently butterbur has been shown to significantly decrease the amount of migraine headaches. I talked to Sally about a placebo-controlled study in which people were given 150 milligrams of butterbur over a four month period and I show her that they had a statistically significant reduction in their migraine headaches in comparison to a placebo group.

I also explained to Sally that butterbur can have liver toxicity. That's why it's very important that, if together we decide this is the right herbal remedy for her, we only use the herbal remedy that was studied and that has a different name, Petadolex. When we pick our herbs, it's important to say, "What herb was used in the study? What parts of the plant? How was it prepared?" so that we have the right formula for the right situation. I recommended butterbur for Sally in the form of Petadolex. I can also tell Sally that 16 randomized controlled trials were reviewed that looked at how well butterbur did next to prescription medications and guess what, prescription medications like inderal, also called propranolol and Topamax were just about as good as butterbur. Said another way, butterbur did as good as the prescription medications in reducing the number of migraine headaches.

Now we have Sally giving up the triggers—the red wine and the cheese. She's thinking about the elimination diet and we're starting to recommend supplements so we have one that has excellent evidence. What else would I recommend at this time? Although they are not herbal remedies, I want to give her all the best that vitamin supplements and herbs have to offer. Number one would be magnesium. Studies have shown a 42 percent reduction in headaches taking just 300 to 400 milligrams of magnesium per day. I will say it throughout this course, magnesium is great because it softens the stool. If someone has constipation, this is an added benefit of magnesium, but if the stool gets too soft I tell my patients you have to cut the magnesium back.

There is equally strong evidence for B vitamin, riboflavin (400 milligrams per day). So now I can recommend to Sally a couple of things, butterbur (150 milligrams in the form of Petadolex), magnesium (300 to 400 milligrams per day), and riboflavin (400 milligrams per day), and there are a few more. We've already talked about the power of omega-3s. Omega-3s are anti inflammatory and omega-3 fish oil is anti inflammatory so I will have Sally take two to four grams per day. In addition, one other supplement has to be mentioned because it statistically reduces migraine headaches and that is CoQ10 300 milligrams per day. Now we have a whole supplement vitamin herbal formula that we can give Sally, but remember Sally is a young woman.

One of the key questions I would ask her before prescribing any herbal remedies or even supplements is does she plan to get pregnant, because, if she plans to get pregnant then I can only use those vitamins, herbs, or supplements that have been proven 100 percent safe in pregnancy. Remember I talked about some supplements that were okay during pregnancy, but not all of them are. In this case, I would say to Sally I feel more comfortable giving you the magnesium, the omega-3 fish oil, and a low dose of the riboflavin because those are the safest choices in case you decide to have a baby. As we have seen, herbs are powerful medicine and because they are powerful medicine, we must be aware of their potential side effects and equally as important herb-drug interactions. Because what I see in my practice is people come in with a shopping bag of vitamin, herbs, and supplements and a shopping bag of pharmaceutical therapies and we need to look at how those two are interacting together.

St. John's Wort is a perfect example of this. Most people know that St. John's Wort helps mild to moderate depression. People go and buy it every day for exactly this reason. It is a great herbal remedy in this situation and we will talk about that in a later lecture. But take a look at what St. John's Wort is capable of doing. If you're taking a medication, like a birth control pill or a heart medicine like digoxin or a blood thinner like Coumadin, this is just a short list. St. John's Wort can decrease the potency of the medications. Even medicines like cyclosporine used for transplants, heart transplants, liver transplants, will be reduced if we add St. John's Wort. Other medications will increase in their potency. Alcohol is amplified in the body when we take St. John's Wort.

It is very important to be aware of herb-drug interactions and there are four categories of prescription medications that I want you to pay particular attention to. These are: blood thinners like Coumadin and souped up aspirins like Plavix and Effient; sedatives, things that relax us, put us to sleep, what we call benzodiazepines, things like valium and Xanax; antidepressants; and diabetes medicine. These four categories are the most common pharmaceutical drugs that we see having herb-drug interactions. If you notice that you're on one of these or in this category, please talk to your physician before starting any natural remedies and you can always get on your computer and go to the naturaldatabase.com website and you can read all about herb, vitamin, and supplement interactions with pharmaceutical therapies or you can go on the FDA website, FDA MedWatch, it's FDA.gov/medwatch for more information.

In closing, I want to leave you with three important points. First, most pharmaceutical drugs come from botanicals so herbal medicine is not alternative medicine. We have seen that herbs are powerful medicine and that they can, when used properly, have a profound effect on our health, but they must be used in the right formulations and in the right doses. When used in this way they can be incredibly effective in treating common, everyday ailments and even more challenging chronic disease.

Lowering Cholesterol Naturally
Lecture 10

The cholesterol-lowering drugs that are so prevalent in the market can reduce the risk of cardiovascular events, but many people are looking for a way to lower their cholesterol without the use of pharmaceuticals. In this lecture, you will learn about cholesterol and the different cholesterol particles. More importantly, you will learn how to impact cholesterol through nutrition, exercise, and supplements. Remember to consult your physician before starting any supplement regimen.

What Is Cholesterol?

- Cholesterol is a waxy substance that is found in the fats in your blood. Your body needs cholesterol to make healthy cells, but having high cholesterol can increase your risk of heart disease.

- Not all cholesterol is bad. In fact, we need to make some important hormones with our cholesterol, such as estrogen for women and testosterone for men.

- All the cholesterol we need is made by the liver. Some people have genetic disorders that lead to high cholesterol, but this is rare. For most of us, high cholesterol is related to our lifestyle. The food we eat, how much alcohol we drink, our physical activity, and even our stress levels play important roles in our cholesterol level.

- Your physician may order a standard blood test to check your cholesterol levels called a lipid panel or a lipid profile. Typical reports include four important numbers: total cholesterol, LDL cholesterol, HDL cholesterol, and triglycerides. These are the four basic components of your cholesterol panel.

- HDL, or high-density lipoprotein, is the good cholesterol. This cholesterol is responsible for pulling plaque out of the arteries.

- LDL, or low-density lipoprotein, is the bad cholesterol. This cholesterol causes plaque in the arteries.

- Having too much LDL (the "lousy" cholesterol) and not enough HDL (the "happy" cholesterol) is what leads to coronary artery disease or a blockage in arteries anywhere in our bodies.

The Truth about Triglycerides

- Triglycerides are a type of fat that circulate in our bloodstream. They store unused calories so that if we go for a long period of time without food, the triglycerides are able to release this energy when we need it.

- Being overweight can increase your triglycerides. Lack of physical activity can also increase triglyceride levels because exercise burns triglycerides. In addition, liquid calories—which are filled with sugar—including alcohol, fruit juice, and soda, contribute to high triglyceride levels. A diet that is high in carbohydrates, especially simple carbohydrates, increase your triglycerides.

- As triglycerides increase, HDL decreases, so if you can lower your triglyceride levels, you can raise the HDL in your body.

- You can take three simple steps—nutrition, exercise, and supplements—to lower your triglyceride levels. Sugar and simple carbohydrates raise the triglycerides. If the triglycerides are high, then the HDL is low.

- The foods that raise triglycerides include simple sugars (cookies, cakes, candy, and ice cream), liquid calories (alcohol, soda, and fruit juice), simple carbohydrates (white bread, white rice, and rice noodles), and starchy vegetables (potatoes and winter squash).

- The best foods to eat are the same foods that will lower your triglycerides, such as whole grains, lentils, and beans. Fruits that are low in sugar—such as apples, peaches, pears, plums, berries, oranges, and grapefruits—can also lower triglyceride levels.

You can also eat green leafy vegetables and omega-3s to lower your triglycerides.

- Two of the best supplements that can be used to lower triglycerides are omega-3 fish oil and the B vitamin niacin.

- Omega-3 fish oil has been shown to decrease triglycerides by 45 percent if you take four grams, or 4,000 milligrams, per day.

- Niacin is not only used to lower triglycerides, but it is also used to raise HDL. Niacin can lower triglycerides by over 50 percent if you take 2,000 milligrams per day.

- However, people with a history of intestinal ulcers, gout, or liver problems should not take niacin. In addition, not all brands of niacin are the same; no-flush niacin does not work to lower the triglycerides or raise the HDL. Niacin should be taken under your physician's guidance because your liver needs to be monitored when taking it.

Lowering the Bad Cholesterol
- Foods that will raise your LDL include saturated fat (beef, pork, lamb, and dark poultry) and full-fat dairy (whole milk, whole cheese, whole cottage cheese, full-fat yogurts, butter, and cream).

- To lower your LDL, substitute the meats you eat with vegetable protein—which has zero cholesterol—and if you consume dairy from a cow, make sure that it is organic and nonfat.

- Organic tofu is a great substitution for meat. Tofu comes from the soybean, so it has no cholesterol. Other options include seitan, which is a flavored wheat product, and tempeh, which is a textured vegetable protein.

- Nuts are a good source of protein, but they are high in calories, so when you eat nuts, use them only as a garnish. In addition, omega-3 eggs can be used to make egg-white omelets, and organic, nonfat yogurt is a great source of protein.

- Fiber can also be used to lower cholesterol. You can find fiber in whole foods such as steel-cut oats and psyllium seeds. Increasing your fiber slowly, you should eventually consume 35 grams of fiber per day.

- Shrimp is a fish that is extremely high in cholesterol. Instead, try to eat wild sockeye salmon or sardines. Both of these are better choices, but fish is still an animal product, and it still contains cholesterol.

Lowering Cholesterol Naturally with Supplements
- Artichoke extract has been shown to lower LDL by 15 percent when taken in a 500-milligram tablet three times per day.

- Taking approximately two grams of plant sterols per day will decrease your LDL by about 10 percent.

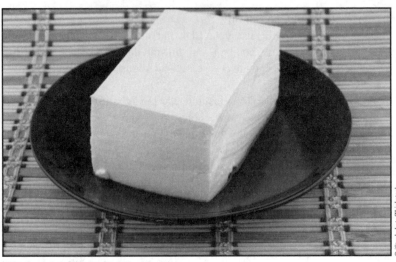

Tofu is a great replacement for chicken in any recipe, and eliminating the chicken eliminates the cholesterol.

- EGCG is the active ingredient of green tea, and taking 500 milligrams of EGCG twice a day will lower your LDL by 13 percent. You can also drink about 60 to 100 ounces per day of organic green tea to get the same effect.

- Taking 300 milligrams of pantothenic acid three times per day can lower your cholesterol as much as 36 percent.

- Red yeast rice, the botanical involved in statin therapy, can be taken in 600-milligram tablets four times per day—two tablets in the morning and two at night for a total of 2,400 milligrams—to reduce cholesterol by 42 percent.

- If you have a history of not being able to take statins (called statin intolerance) or if you have muscle or joint aches, do not take red yeast rice as a supplement. Red yeast rice can also lower the enzyme CoQ10, so when taking red yeast rice, also take 100 milligrams per day of CoQ10.

Questions to Consider

1. What are HDL and LDL?

2. Which foods raise cholesterol, and which foods raise triglycerides?

Lowering Cholesterol Naturally
Lecture 10—Transcript

Welcome back. You see commercials all the time about cholesterol lowering medication. Commercials touting the virtues of drugs like Zocor and Lipitor. And it is true, these cholesterol lowering drugs can reduce the risk of cardiovascular events. But many people, especially my patients, can't or do not want to take these medications. Like many of my patients they are looking for a way to lower their cholesterol without the use of pharmaceuticals. In other words, people are looking for ways to lower their cholesterol naturally. Is this even possible? Well I can tell you unequivocally that the answer is yes!

Today we will learn about cholesterol and the different cholesterol particles. More importantly we will learn how to impact cholesterol through nutrition, exercise, and supplements. But first, we have to ask a question. What is cholesterol and where does it come from? Cholesterol is a waxy substance that is found in the fats in your blood. Your body needs cholesterol to make healthy cells, but having high cholesterol can increase your risk of heart disease. So, not all cholesterol is bad. In fact, we need to make some really important hormones with our cholesterol; like estrogen for women and testosterone for men.

So where does cholesterol come from? Well, all the cholesterol we ever need is made by the liver. We never have to say, "Let me go out and have a high cholesterol meal so I can make some healthy cells or I can make my sex hormones like estrogen and testosterone." Some people have genetic disorders that lead to high cholesterol, but this is rare. For most of us, high cholesterol is related to our lifestyle. The food we eat, how much alcohol we drink, our physical activity, and even stress play important roles in our cholesterol level.

Your physician may order a standard blood test, a blood test to check your cholesterol levels; this is called a lipid panel or a lipid profile. Typical reports include four important numbers. First a lipid panel will have a total cholesterol; number two, an LDL cholesterol; number three, HDL cholesterol; and number four, triglycerides. These are the four components or basic components of your cholesterol panel. Let's look at some of these a little closer. HDL stands for high density lipoprotein. This is the good cholesterol. This cholesterol is responsible for pulling plaque out of the arteries. My patients taught me that the H in HDL is for the happy cholesterol.

LDL stands for low density lipoprotein. Guess what the L stands for. You got it! My patients call that the lousy cholesterol, the cholesterol that we frequently say causes plaque in the arteries. But, the reality is too little HDL, too little of the good stuff, too much of the bad stuff, the LDL, that is what leads to coronary artery disease or blockage in arteries anywhere in our bodies. So let us take a look at the other component of our lipid profile, called triglycerides.

Triglycerides are a type of fat that circulate in our bloodstream. They actually store unused calories so that if we go for a long period of time without food the triglycerides are able to release this energy when we need it. Let's begin. Let's start with triglycerides first. Let's talk about where they come from and then what we can do to lower them. I teach it to my patients this way. Triglycerides come from a couple of important places. First, just being overweight—just having extra weight in your midline can increase your triglycerides. Second, lack of physical activity—when we exercise or we decide to walk up the steps instead of taking the elevator we burn triglycerides. The liquid calories—we have three liquid calories that are filled with sugar: alcohol, fruit juice, and soda. And the fourth is a diet that is high in carbohydrates, especially simple carbohydrates (the white stuff).

Now there is one important thing I need to emphasize about triglycerides. They keep company with the good cholesterol, HDL. I tell my patients it is like a seesaw, as triglycerides go up, the good cholesterol, the HDL, goes down. If we can bring down the triglycerides—that's right—we raise the HDL. The question is, how do we lower the triglycerides naturally?

It comes down to three simple steps, nutrition, exercise, and supplements. Let's always start where I like to begin: food first. Sugar and simple carbohydrates raise our triglycerides. As a matter of fact, I use the same nutrition program to lower triglycerides as I do to prevent and treat diabetes. But remember, that is not all. If the triglycerides are high, the HDL, the good cholesterol, is low and that HDL is what we need to pull plaque out of the artery. The foods that raise triglycerides you already know. Simple sugar, cookies, cakes, candy, and ice cream, we mention the liquid calories alcohol, soda, and fruit juice and the simple carbohydrates will raise triglycerides, white bread, white rice, rice noodles, and an Italian favorite called gnocchi. This is a potato pasta guaranteed to raise your triglycerides. Now starchy vegetables will also raise triglycerides—things like potatoes and winter squash.

You already know the best foods to eat, and these same foods will lower your triglycerides; foods like whole grains, lentils, and beans. When we pick a fruit, let's pick a fruit that is low in sugar like apples, peach, pear, plums, and berries. Even oranges and grapefruits, when we eat them whole, will not raise our triglycerides. And of course, my absolute favorite are the green leafy vegetables and we can add in some omega-3s like wild salmon or sardines if you like them.

Now I have two favorite supplements that I like to use to lower triglycerides. So once I have convinced my patients that they are going to change their diet, they are cleaning out the pantry, cleaning out the refrigerator, all the white stuff and liquid calories are going, we are going to talk a bit about exercise, the next thing I do is I say, What are the two supplements I can use? My two favorites are omega-3 fish oil and the B vitamin niacin.

You may recall from the talk on vitamins and supplements that I mentioned omega-3 fish oil. Omega-3 fish oil has been shown to decrease triglycerides 45 percent if you take four grams. That is 4000 milligrams or four grams of omega-3 fish oil can decrease triglycerides 45 percent. Now that is powerful medicine. So what about our second supplement, niacin? Niacin is one of the tried and true vitamins for lowering triglycerides. It is also used, as you can imagine, to raise HDL. So it is also the magic vitamin for raising the good cholesterol, but no surprise because of the seesaw effect, triglycerides go down, HDL goes up, 2000 milligrams of niacin per day can lower triglycerides over 50 percent.

But there are some really important caveats about niacin that you need to know before you decide to go and buy this vitamin. People with a history of intestinal ulcers, gout, or liver problems should not take niacin. Number two, not all brands of niacin are the same. You will see on the shelf things that say "no-flush niacin"; these frequently do not work to lower the triglycerides or raise the HDL. Number three, niacin is one of those vitamins that I really want you to take under your physician's guidance because we need to monitor your liver when we give you niacin. So now, we know how to lower triglycerides and raise HDL and I promise you, if you have high triglycerides, and you give up all the white stuff and start to walk every day, you are going to really impress your physician when you have your next blood test.

Let's now turn our attention to the LDL, the so called "bad" (or what my patients call the "lousy") cholesterol. Let's start with food first. Well this is the way I teach it to my patients. I say if it has a smiling face, two eyes, it has cholesterol. That means cholesterol comes from animals. What foods will raise your LDL cholesterol? What foods will raise the so called bad cholesterol? You know these: saturated fat, things like beef, pork, and lamb. Dark poultry, like dark turkey and dark chicken meat are another source of saturated fat. Full fat dairy, full fat or whole milk, whole cheeses, whole cottage cheese, full fat yogurts, all of these will raise your LDL cholesterol. And of course butter and cream will raise your LDL cholesterol.

Now you already know I want you to read the labels and if you have to buy something in a package please make sure it does not contain trans fats or partially hydrogenated oils, and of course, you already know it shouldn't contain high fructose corn syrup, which is sugar. Rule number one for lowering your LDL; more vegetable protein and if you have dairy from a cow it has to be organic and nonfat, and we will talk more about organic in a later lecture. Remember cholesterol only comes from animals, so let's start to make some substitutions. You might say what am I going to eat for my beef, my pork, my lamb, my dark meat chicken, my dark meat turkey, what is Dr. G. going to have me eat?

Well vegetable protein is a good start because vegetable protein has zero cholesterol. That is right, zero cholesterol. In fact, if you can identify a food as coming from the earth it has zero cholesterol. There are some high fat foods that come from the earth that we eat small amounts of. We talked about some of these, like nuts, olives, and olive oil, the good monounsaturated fats, eat small amounts of those. But if you can identify it coming from the earth, you can be certain that it has no cholesterol. So instead of that beef, pork, and lamb let's try some more beans, more lentils, and more legumes, zero cholesterol.

You might even want to branch out to some different items, things you may be less familiar with; organic tofu is a great choice. Tofu comes from the soybean, no cholesterol. Then there are two others, one is called seitan and the other is tempeh, a textured vegetable protein. The good news about this is when I make it at my house, no one knows the difference. I do not think they know if they are eating meat or if they are eating tofu or if they are eating seitan because it all works out the same. Tofu is a great replacement for chicken in any recipe, and cutting out the chicken cuts out the cholesterol.

In an earlier lecture, I talked about another source of protein, which is nuts. Now nuts are a good source of protein, but remember they are high in calories so when you have your nuts you have 15 nuts, because as we said that is about 170 to 180 calories so use the nuts as a garnish. One of the tricks I like to use with my patients to get them some extra protein is to make a protein smoothie, so in the morning they can take almond milk or rice milk or even their organic fat free milk and they can add two scoops of a good protein and they can add some organic berries and that gives them an extra protein pickup in the morning. Omega-3, eggs can be used to make egg white omelets and of course yogurt, good organic nonfat yogurt, is a great choice of protein.

Now do not forget my favorite, fiber. We have talked a lot about fiber in previous lectures. I use fiber to lower cholesterol everywhere. I use it as a supplement because you can buy fiber as a supplement or I like to use it as a food. Fiber lowers cholesterol. I have patients in my practice who have lowered their cholesterol 50 to 70 points just by adding in fiber. Remember, you find the fiber in whole foods like steel cut oats. One ounce of steel cut oats has three grams of fiber. Our goal is to eat 35 grams of fiber per day. And remember what I said in the previous lecture. Do not eat the fiber all at once because if you are not used to fiber it can cause a lot of gas and a lot of bloating so increase your fiber slowly, knowing that your goal is 35 grams per day.

You may want to buy some psyllium, psyllium seeds, and you can sprinkle that on your steel cut oats because one tablespoon has anywhere from five to seven grams of fiber. Read your labels. Only buy those foods that are high fiber foods if you are buying anything in a package. What about fish? Well, the two things you need to know are this. Shrimp, which I know a lot of people like are extremely high in cholesterol and my people, the Italians, love a fish called calamari, which is very high in cholesterol. It is high in cholesterol before you even deep fry it making it a really bad food for your heart, for your brain and everything else. So buy some wild sockeye salmon, you can even buy it in a can; or sardines if you enjoy sardines. These are your better choices, but remember fish is still an animal product and it still contains cholesterol.

Now that we know what to eat to lower cholesterol, now that we are going to add more whole foods and vegetarian protein into our diet, what supplements can you take so that we can continue to lower our cholesterol naturally? Well I have a list of supplements that is really long, but I am going to give you only a few of my superstars today. We already talked about the B vitamin niacin, lowering triglycerides, raising the good cholesterol HDL. We already talked about fish oil, the omega-3s for lowering triglycerides. Remember, four grams per day of omega-3 lowers triglycerides 45 percent. Now we want to go after the LDL, the so called "bad" cholesterol.

What can we do? Now, I have these supplements numbered, but this does not mean I prefer one over the other. I like them all, and sometimes I will use something different for one individual and something else for someone else. All of these are good for lowering the LDL. The first is a supplement called Artichoke Extract. Artichoke Extract has been studied and has been shown to lower the LDL 15 percent when taken in a 500 milligram tablet three times a day. Artichoke Extract is a good choice for many of my patients.

Number two, something called plant sterols. Remember we talked about plants having a lot of healing properties. Well sterols are one of them. When we eat plant sterols the body looks at it as if it is cholesterol. It almost looks like the cholesterol particle so it blocks the cholesterol from getting into our bloodstream because it sits on the same receptors so plant sterols block cholesterol absorption. If you take them two to 2.5 grams a day they will decrease your LDL around 10 percent. Sometimes I like to have my patients add those plant sterols to their smoothie. There are even smoothies on the market that contain plant sterols in them.

The third supplement I like to use is called EGCG. This is the active ingredient of green tea. If you take this, 500 milligrams of EGCG two times a day you will lower your LDL, the bad cholesterol 13 percent. Now you might say to me, "I enjoy drinking green tea, can't I drink it Dr. G.?" Absolutely, drink organic green tea, but you have to drink about 60 to 100 ounces a day, so I tell my patients their two drinks throughout the day should be filtered water, remember not out of a plastic bottle, and organic green tea, and please do not buy a bottle that says green tea that has sugar added to it, because that will defeat the purpose.

What other supplements do we have? Well number four is pantothenic acid. Pantothenic acid has been well researched and when taken 300 milligrams three times a day can lower cholesterol as much as 36 percent. That is huge, that is as much as any statin therapy on the market, so this is a good choice if you decide I want to take a supplement to lower my cholesterol. Then my last one; number five, red yeast rice. I have to separate this out from the others because red yeast rice is the botanical that gives us statin therapy, so it is very important. If you have a history of not being able to take statins, what we call statin intolerance, muscle aches, joint aches, if your physician has taken you off of a statin because you have a side effect to it, do not run out and start taking high doses of red yeast rice because you can have the same side effects, but red yeast rice at 2400 milligrams a day, usually it comes in 600 milligram tablets, I have my patients take two in the morning and two at night, will lower cholesterol 42 percent.

And just like a statin I am concerned that red yeast rice can lower the enzyme called CoQ10, which is an important enzyme for the power of our cells so when I give red yeast rice I also give Coenzyme Q10 100 milligrams per day. Remember when you decide to go on a supplement regimen to consult your physician before starting any supplement, and what I tell my patients is this; do not expect to lower your cholesterol, your triglycerides, your LDL, do not expect any changes if you are still going to go around and eat beef, pork, and lamb, and throw cream in your coffee, and have cheese and all the saturated fat that we talked about, because that is just defeating the purpose.

Today we reviewed the foods and supplements that lower cholesterol. At the end of the day I can assure you we do not have to rely on big pharma to get our cholesterol profile perfect. We have the tools to lower our cholesterol naturally and I invite you to take the first steps to do so.

Treating High Blood Pressure Naturally
Lecture 11

In addition to cholesterol, another major risk factor for heart disease and stroke is high blood pressure, which is also known as hypertension. High blood pressure is often referred to as "the silent killer" because most people are unaware that they have high blood pressure. In this lecture, you will learn about the natural ways to treat high blood pressure by addressing four key components: nutrition, exercise, supplements, and responses to stress and tension.

What Is Blood Pressure?

- Blood pressure is the force of blood exerted against the walls of the arteries in your body. It is measured in millimeters of mercury and is recorded as two numbers. The top number is called the systolic blood pressure, which is the number that assesses the pressure when the heart squeezes. The bottom number is the diastolic blood pressure, which is the number that assesses the pressure when the heart rests. Both numbers are equally important.

- Before the age of 55, it appears in the research that the diastolic blood pressure is a greater predictor of future cardiovascular events, or future risks. After the age of 55, the top number, the systolic blood pressure, predicts risk the best.

- A normal blood pressure is 120/80. If you have a blood pressure between 120 and 139 on the top or between 80 and 89 on the bottom, then you are considered to have prehypertension. If your blood pressure is 140/90 or above, you have high blood pressure.

Decreasing Blood Pressure Naturally

- The best way to decrease your blood pressure naturally is to decrease your weight. Eleven clinical trials have shown that for every one kilogram of weight that is lost, the systolic blood pressure is decreased by 1.6 millimeters of mercury and the diastolic blood pressure is decreased by 1.1 millimeters of mercury.

- A body composition tells you how much fat you have on your body and how much muscle you have on your body. Ideally, women should have a body fat composition of less than 22 and men should have a body fat composition of less than 16.

- The best ways to decrease your weight are proper nutrition and exercise. Combining daily aerobic exercise (40 minutes to one hour per day) with strength training (three times per week) has been shown to decrease blood pressure by 10 to 15 millimeters of mercury on the top and five to 10 millimeters of mercury on the bottom.

- Exercise is medicine. It increases lean muscle mass, burns calories, and decreases your weight—which decreases your blood pressure. Exercise lowers your triglycerides, blood sugar, and LDL cholesterol. Exercise also helps mentally; it is a treatment for depression and anxiety.

- Alcohol raises blood pressure, and when you drink alcohol, you also tend to eat more. Alcohol is sugar and should be restricted.

- One cup of coffee per day, which has about 100 milligrams of caffeine, is the maximum that you can drink if you want to get your blood pressure down. Organic green tea is a much better choice, with only 20 milligrams of caffeine.

- Sodium, or salt, is one of the major issues with the standard American diet. The average American takes in about 5,000 milligrams of sodium per day, but the body only needs 500 milligrams. There is a direct relationship between sodium intake and blood pressure.

- Salt is in packaged and canned foods. Salt is also hidden in just about every item on a menu at a restaurant. Look for the sodium content on the label of any packaged or canned foods that you buy, and keep your sodium content under 1,500 milligrams per day.

- Research shows that if you replace high omega-6 oils—such as corn oil, safflower oil, and sunflower oil—with extra virgin olive oil, you can lower your blood pressure by about eight millimeters of mercury.

- Garlic lowers blood pressure. Four cloves of fresh garlic every day will lower your systolic blood pressure by 10 points. You will get the same benefit as four cloves of garlic per day in 900 milligrams of aged garlic extract.

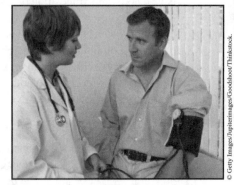

By exercising, you can decrease your weight, which will result in lower blood pressure.

- Consuming about three grams per day of high-quality, dried wakame, or seaweed, will lower your blood pressure by 14 millimeters of mercury on the top.

- Drinking 30 grams of hydrolyzed whey protein in a smoothie every day can reduce your systolic blood pressure by 11 points.

- Lycopene, the active ingredient in tomatoes, has been proven to lower blood pressure. Enjoy fresh tomatoes or take a lycopene supplement.

Micronutrients and Supplements
- Magnesium—which we need for our bones, heart, and bowel functions—is a mineral that can be obtained by consuming green leafy vegetables, but 68 percent of U.S. adults consume less than the recommended daily allowance.

- Research shows that as the intracellular level of magnesium, or the red blood cell magnesium, decreases, blood pressure increases. Supplementing magnesium will lower your blood pressure about five millimeters of mercury on the top and about three on the bottom.

- If you decide to use magnesium as a supplement, there are three beneficial preparations: chelated magnesium, magnesium aspartate, and magnesium glycinate. Take about 500 milligrams per day of any of these. People with kidney problems should not take magnesium without a physician's guidance.

- People with low levels of vitamin D tend to have the highest blood pressure. The lower your 25-hydroxy vitamin D, the higher your blood pressure. Vitamin D supplementation—with or without a vitamin D deficiency—has been shown in both animals and humans (both men and women) to decrease blood pressure.

- Research has shown that vitamin D replacement decreases blood pressure approximately 13 points on the top. A 25-hydroxy vitamin D level that is above 55 is ideal and appears to protect against breast cancer in women. Vitamin D can be taken in high doses, such as about 10,000 international units per day.

- Another deficiency that is associated with high blood pressure is the deficiency of enzyme CoQ10. The lower the CoQ10, the higher the blood pressure. Research shows that taking 200 to 400 milligrams of CoQ10 per day can lower systolic blood pressure by 11 points.

- Adding more omega-3s (fish) and eliminating saturated fats can also help you lower your blood pressure. Research shows that four grams of omega-3 per day will lower blood pressure by around eight millimeters of mercury.

- In addition to micronutrients and supplements, dealing with the stress in your life in a calm manner can help lower your blood pressure. Stress causes blood pressure to rise, so the next time you are experiencing stress or tension, take a deep breath and react calmly.

Questions to Consider

1. Limiting sodium to how many milligrams per day lowers blood pressure significantly?

2. A 10-kg weight loss will reduce systolic blood pressure by how many mm Hg?

Treating High Blood Pressure Naturally
Lecture 11—Transcript

In our last lecture we discussed cholesterol and we said it is a major risk factor for heart disease. Another major risk factor for heart disease and stroke is high blood pressure, also known as hypertension. In medicine we call high blood pressure the silent killer because most people are unaware that they even have high blood pressure. Today, we will discuss natural ways to treat high blood pressure. The four key components to treating high blood pressure naturally are: 1) nutrition; 2) exercise; 3) supplements; and 4) how we change our response to stress and tension.

Let's start by asking the question, "What is blood pressure?" Blood pressure is the force of blood exerted against the walls of our arteries. It is measured in millimeters of mercury and recorded as two numbers. The top number is called the systolic blood pressure. That is when the heart beats, when it squeezes. The bottom number is the diastolic blood pressure, when the heart rests. Both numbers are equally important.

Before the age of 55, it appears in the research that the diastolic blood pressure is a greater predictor of future cardiovascular events, in other words, a future risk. After the age of 55 the top number, the systolic blood pressure, predicts risk the best. Let's review what a normal blood pressure is. A normal blood pressure is 120/80. If you have a blood pressure between 120 and 139 on the top or between 80 and 89 on the bottom you are considered to have pre-hypertension. If your blood pressure is 140/90 or above, you already have high blood pressure.

The first thing I tell my patients, the best way to decrease your blood pressure naturally is to decrease your weight. I can't overemphasize this. Eleven clinical trials have shown for every one kilogram of weight that we lose, we decrease the systolic blood pressure 1.6 millimeters of mercury. For every one kilogram of weight we lose we decrease the diastolic blood pressure by 1.1 millimeters of mercury. Let's take a look at this. We decide to lose 10 kilograms; that is 22 pounds, we would decrease the top number of our blood pressure, the systolic blood pressure by 16 points and we would decrease the bottom number by 10 points. There is only one medicine that is going to give us that and this medicine is called weight loss.

We want you to get a body composition. A body composition tells me how much fat you have on your body and how much muscle you have on your body. This is even more important than getting on the scale. For women, we want a body fat composition less than 22 and for men less than 16.

You know the way to decrease your weight: proper nutrition and exercise. These are the best ways to decrease your weight. Regular aerobic exercise daily with strength training has been shown to decrease blood pressure 10 to 15 millimeters of mercury on the top and five to 10 millimeters of mercury on the bottom. On average, if we can get you trained and get you moving and get you fit, we can decrease the top number of your blood pressure 11 points.

What I tell my patients is this: "You eat everyday so guess what? You have to exercise every day." The Council of Clinical Cardiology is very clear with their recommendations: aerobic exercise—things like walking, and swimming, and jogging, and treadmill, and biking, anything that gets us going—every day of the week, 40 minutes to one hour. Strength training, light weights, multiple repetitions, at least three times per week. These are the minimal recommendations for exercise. Exercise is medicine. There is not a thing that exercise does not improve. Exercise increases lean muscle mass. We get more muscle. We get rid of that extra fat when we exercise. Exercise burns calories and decreases our weight. And remember, decreasing weight decreases blood pressure.

Exercise also helps us mentally. Believe it or not exercise is a treatment for depression and for anxiety. We have talked about cholesterol. Well, guess what? Exercise will lower your triglycerides, will lower your blood sugar, and will even lower your LDL cholesterol. So exercise is a key component to reducing your blood pressure.

What about food? You already know the right things to eat. Let's review a few. Again, number one, whole foods; you will get tired of me saying this. Every time you pick up an apple you will say Dr. G. fresh fruit and veggies get those green leafy vegetables on your plate. Whole grains, like steel cut oats, remember fiber lowers cholesterol. What else? Plant-based protein, more beans, more lentils, more tofu, use nuts (again, as a garnish), and our omega-3 fish. These are sort of the basics, if you might, of our nutritional foundation.

Now there is something I have to tell you that most people do not like to hear. I need you to restrict your alcohol. Alcohol raises blood pressure. Most people know this, when you drink you tend to eat more. What my patients tell me is, "By the second drink Dr. G., I am not worried about my diet anymore; I figure I will worry about that tomorrow." So alcohol restriction is important when it comes to blood pressure and of course you know alcohol is sugar. It is liquid calories.

What about caffeine? One cup of coffee a day is the max if you want to get your blood pressure down. One cup coffee has about 100 milligrams of caffeine so you would do better if you took your caffeine in the form of organic green tea. That has only 20 milligrams of caffeine, a much better choice. But when it comes to blood pressure we need to address the role of sodium, of salt. This is one of the major issues we have with the standard American diet. The average American takes in about 5000 milligrams of sodium per day. Some people, do not ask me how, can consume 15 to 20,000 milligrams of sodium per day, yet the body only needs 500 milligrams. The body does not need this kind of sodium and just like with weight there is a direct relationship between your sodium intake and your blood pressure. This has been proven.

The National Heart, Lung, and Blood Institute did an amazing study. The institute looked at a diet called the DASH II diet, and they said let's take people on the standard American diet, and if you have not caught onto it yet the acronym is SAD, and they said those people can eat what typical Americans eat, over 3000 milligrams of sodium a day. And then they said let's restrict the sodium a little bit. Let's get an intermediate group of 2300 milligrams of sodium a day and then let's get really creative and let's take the sodium and drop it down to 1500 milligrams per day, three groups. Now remember the body only needs how much, 500 milligrams of sodium, so the body is getting three times what it needs anyway.

These studies clearly show the benefit of sodium reduction. In the DASH II Diet, people who had high blood pressure eating 1500 milligrams of sodium per day were able to drop their blood pressure 11.5 points on the top and 6.8 points on the bottom. That is the difference between needing blood pressure medicine and not needing blood pressure medicine. For this reason, based on this research and many years of clinical practice, I tell my patients I want you on a less than 1500 milligram per day sodium diet.

Many of my patients said to me, "Dr. G., I never use the salt shaker. I do not touch it. We do not have it in the house, I swear." I tell them I believe them, I believe they are not using the salt shaker, but the salt is in packaged and canned foods. For people that eat in restaurants salt is hidden in just about everything.

Did you know that just three ounces of ham—and you know I do not want you to eat ham anyway—has 1000 milligrams of sodium? One little cup of canned chicken noodle soup has 1400 milligrams of sodium. Now that is not even the entire can. There is more than one cup in a can, so if you decide to have that one cup of chicken noodle soup you already have all your sodium for the day. Two slices of white bread—which I know you won't eat anymore—has 340 milligrams of sodium. On the other hand, remember our friend whole foods? One cup of almonds, unsalted—the unsalted is important here—one milligram of sodium. And a mango, a whole mango five milligrams of sodium. You only find sodium in a package or a can.

Remember, read your labels. Look for the sodium on the label, but also look where it says serving size. This is one of the great tricks of the food industry. They may say there is only 500 milligrams of sodium, but then you look at the serving size and you find wow that's in one ounce so if I have four ounces I have 2000 milligrams of sodium. So, read the labels and keep the sodium less than 1500 milligrams per day. You will see a marked reduction in your blood pressure. Combine that with your weight loss, combine that with your exercise and you are going to see a huge difference.

Clearly, lowering your sodium intake is one of the key things that you can do to lower your blood pressure. The research proves it, and I see it every day in my practice. What else can we do? Well you have heard me talk a lot about extra virgin olive oil. Well the research shows that if you replace the high omega-6 oils like corn oil, safflower oil, and sunflower oil with extra virgin olive oil you can lower your blood pressure about eight millimeters of mercury. I do not want you to use those other oils anyway. Stick with the extra virgin olive oil.

What about garlic? Not everyone likes garlic, but for those of us that do garlic lowers blood pressure. Four cloves of fresh garlic everyday will lower your systolic blood pressure 10 points. Now your spouse or your partner may not want you eating that garlic, and I can understand why, unless they eat it as well. In that case you may want to take aged garlic extract. You will get the same benefit as four cloves of garlic per day in 900 milligrams of aged garlic extract.

Another good one, really good one, for lowering blood pressure is seaweed. Now before you rush off and go and buy seaweed I do not want you to buy the kind that comes in a bag as a snack, what is it covered in? It is covered in salt and partially hydrogenated oils. I want you to get the high quality, dried wakame, 3.3 grams per day. This will lower blood pressure 14 millimeters of mercury on the top. That is pretty powerful medicine. So we have extra virgin olive oil, we have garlic, there is a great dish for you by the way, broccoli, garlic, and some extra virgin olive oil that you put on afterwards, perfect dish. Seaweed, 3.3 grams of the dried wakame a day, and for my patients who like smoothies, I recommend a hydrolyzed whey protein smoothie. Hydrolyzed whey protein goes through a special process, 30 grams which is usually depending on the brand, one or two scoops, 30 grams in a smoothie everyday can reduce systolic blood pressure 11 points.

Remember we talked about protein coming in the form of a smoothie to give us that extra boost that we need. So these are just some of the few really good food choices that can impact our blood pressure, and there is one more. Remember our friend the tomato, another one of those great whole foods. Well lycopene, the active ingredient in tomatoes has been tested. In an extract form, which means in a pill or capsule form, the active ingredient in tomatoes also lowers blood pressure. So enjoy your tomatoes and if you want, you can take a lycopene supplement.

We have discussed the role of weight loss, we talked about exercise, a low sodium diet, and some really good foods for treating high blood pressure. Next we will shift gears and take a look at some of the micronutrients and supplements that we should also consider. But just in review, remember one kilogram of weight loss decreases systolic blood pressure 1.6 millimeters of mercury. If you lose that 10 kilograms we can decrease blood pressure by 16 points and after this lecture, I expect no one to eat more than 1500 milligrams of sodium per day if you have high blood pressure.

Let's go and look at the micronutrients and the supplements. You will hear me say this over and over again. My favorite mineral is magnesium, yet 68 percent of U.S. adults, consume less than the recommended daily allowance. Where do we get magnesium from? We get magnesium from our green leafy vegetables, our dark greens. We need magnesium for our bones. We need magnesium for our heart, and without magnesium we probably would not have a bowel movement.

The research shows that as the intracellular level of magnesium goes down, blood pressure goes up. Now many people will go to their physician and say measure my magnesium level and the physician measures what is called a serum magnesium. Do not fall for this trap. If you decide you want your magnesium level checked, you tell your physician, "I want an intracellular magnesium or a red blood cell magnesium." That is really what tells us what is going on with your magnesium inside the cell. Another option is to just supplement. Magnesium will lower blood pressure somewhere in the range of five millimeters of mercury on the top and about three on the bottom.

Now you may say, "Well that is not a lot Dr. G.," but magnesium has so many other good benefits. For people with skipped or extra heart beats, I use magnesium all the time. Remember I said it is great for constipation so if you tend to run a little bit on the constipated side magnesium for you is a homerun. If you decide to use magnesium as a supplement there are one of three preparations that I would like you to take. One would be called chelated magnesium, and it will say this right on the bottle. The second is magnesium aspartate and the third is magnesium glycinate. I usually prescribe around 500 milligrams per day, but I do not give that dose all at one. Maybe I will give 250 milligrams a day to start because if someone is sensitive they may end up with soft stool. If someone says I have a lot of constipation I may push the magnesium levels up to as high as 1000 milligrams per day. Now your physician will want to give you prescription magnesium. It's called magnesium oxide. This one is notorious for causing stomach pain and that's why I don't recommend it. There is on important caveat about magnesium. People with kidney problems, people who have renal disease or kidney failure, should not take magnesium without their physician's guidance.

Now let's take a look at a vitamin. We took a look at a mineral, magnesium. Now let's take a look at vitamin D. We know that people with low levels of vitamin D tend to have the highest blood pressure, a very similar relationship that we see with magnesium. Remember we said if the intracellular magnesium is low the blood pressure is high. We see the same thing with vitamin D. The lower your 25-hydroxy vitamin D, by the way that is the blood test you want to have, 25-hydroxy vitamin D, the lower the vitamin D the higher the blood pressure. Vitamin D supplementation with or without even a vitamin D deficiency has been shown in both animals and humans to decrease blood pressure. This is true in both men and in women.

One very interesting study, called the Pfeiffer Women's Study, showed vitamin D replacement decreased blood pressure 13 points on the top. When you go and get your blood tested you tell your physician, "I want a 25-hydroxy vitamin D." What I want you to do with the information is know that our goal is to get your level above 55. A serum level around 55 to 60 is just perfect, and also appears to protect against breast cancer in women. Now vitamin D can be taken in high doses and we do not really think that it is toxic in doses about 10,000 international units per day, but get your level checked and let your physician guide your replacements.

There is one third deficiency that is associated with high blood pressure. This is deficiency of an enzyme called CoQ10. CoQ10 is used by the energy producing component in our cell, called the mitochondria, to make energy. If we do not have CoQ10 we have no energy. CoQ10 deficiency has been linked to high blood pressure just like with vitamin D, the lower the CoQ10, and, yes, you can get your level measured, the lower the CoQ10, the higher the blood pressure. So how do we get CoQ10 deficiency? Well it happens as we get older; somehow we start to deplete ourselves of CoQ10. Usually that is because we have some other chronic diseases, like heart disease or high blood pressure or diabetes. A common cause of CoQ10 deficiency is statin therapy. Statin medications, as you have already heard, given to lower cholesterol also deplete the body of CoQ10. What the research shows us is that CoQ10 taken 200 to 400 milligrams a day can lower systolic blood pressure 11 points.

So we have a few things we need to consider when we are talking about supplements. Magnesium, what is my intracellular magnesium, or just take it. CoQ10, add that into your regimen, and of course vitamin D. These are all important, easy to get, easy to check, simple solutions to helping treat high blood pressure. Last but not least, you have heard me mention omega-3 many times already. Get rid of your saturated fat and add more fish into your diet and you know I even want you to add more of the vegetable protein, the bean, the lentils, and legumes, but the research does show that omega-3 supplementation, here comes that magic number again, four grams, remember we said four grams lowers triglycerides, four grams of omega-3 will lower you blood pressure around eight millimeters of mercury. That is another good choice for treating high blood pressure naturally.

Let's review. We discussed the first thing, the first, number one for decreasing blood pressure is decreasing our weight. We need to work on that immediately. How do we get there? Number two, exercise, aerobic exercise, 40 minutes to one hour a day every single day and if you say you want to take a Sabbath and not exercise one day I will say okay I will let you go six days a week. Strength training, three times a week, this will significantly decrease your blood pressure. Now let's add something on top of that. We are losing weight, we are exercising, we are cleaning out the cupboards, we are done with sodium, less than 1500 milligrams per day. That means getting rid of packaged and canned foods nine out of 10 times; you have to read those labels. Talk to your physician about some of the supplements that we discussed today.

There is a fifth thing you can do. We will talk about it at length in future lectures, but remember for now when you feel stressed take a deep breath. This will help to lower your blood pressure, but before we get to that our next lecture we will discuss natural approaches to diabetes.

Treating Diabetes Naturally
Lecture 12

In this lecture, you will learn about a spectrum of sugar, or metabolism, disorders that range from prediabetes to full-blown diabetes. You're not going to learn about the kind of diabetes that occurs early in life as a result of pancreatic failure; instead, you're going to learn about the kind of diabetes that results from lifestyle—including what kind of food you eat, how physically active you are, and how you respond to stress and tension. You will also discover the tools that can help you prevent and even reverse diabetes.

The Diabetes Spectrum

- Diabetes is one of the key risk factors for kidney disease, leading to dialysis, heart disease, and stroke. Diabetes affects every organ in the body.

- We need to think of the diagnosis of diabetes as the end result of a much longer continuum—starting with insulin resistance and metabolic syndrome before manifesting the disease known as diabetes. This is important because even before the blood tests show that you have diabetes, there are signs that can be attended to.

- One of the first signs that you are at risk for developing diabetes is the presence of insulin resistance. Insulin is a hormone that controls blood sugar and is produced by the pancreas. Stimuli such as insulin and even exercise carry blood sugar into the cells, where they can use it for energy.

- Insulin resistance occurs when the transport of sugar into the cell no longer works properly. The pancreas has to keep working harder and harder to produce more insulin, and eventually, the pancreas can't keep up. It becomes exhausted and can't produce enough insulin. This is when people develop insulin-requiring diabetes and need insulin injections.

- Insulin resistance is part of a larger syndrome called metabolic syndrome, which has four components: insulin resistance, high blood pressure, abnormalities in the cholesterol panel (low HDL and high triglycerides), and abdominal obesity (wearing your weight in the midline).

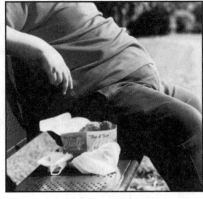

Obesity is often associated with insulin resistance, which results in having problems controlling blood-sugar levels.

- Nearly 27 percent of adults in the United States are obese—that's 72 million Americans. By the end of the decade, it is predicted that the annual cost for diabetes and prediabetes alone will be 500 billion dollars.

- There are five key areas that people on the path to diabetes need to focus on: proper nutrition, physical activity, responses to stress and tension, sleep patterns, and environmental toxins.

- Most people don't realize that lack of sleep can lead to insulin resistance. Lack of sleep is a stress on the body, and stress raises blood sugar and makes insulin resistance worse. Research shows that people who tend to get five hours or less of sleep each night have a higher risk of developing diabetes.

Preventing and Reversing Diabetes: Nutrition
- Nutrition is the key to shifting the diabetes continuum. Sugar and carbohydrates are digested at different rates, and the rate of digestion is called the glycemic index. The higher the index, the faster the body converts food to sugar.

- Another way of measuring the conversion of food to sugar is called the glycemic load, which is an even more accurate assessment of the impact of food on blood sugar and, ultimately, on insulin levels.

- A food with a glycemic load of greater than 20 is high, and a food with a glycemic load of less than 10 is low. Foods that have a low glycemic index and a low glycemic load are the foods that are the best for everyone, but especially for someone who is overweight, prediabetic, or has diabetes.

- In general, you should not eat foods that spike up your insulin level. Insulin has been linked to cancers and leads to inflammation.

- Soluble fiber—which is found in oats, bran, beans, and lentils—lowers cholesterol and blood sugar. Green leafy vegetables have a very low glycemic load and low glycemic index. Cruciferous vegetables, such as cauliflower, broccoli, and cabbage, are all good choices. Other options include omega-3 eggs and omega-3 fish, such as salmon, mackerel, anchovies, sardines, and herring. Lean meat such as free-range chicken and turkey will not spike up your insulin.

- Choose fruits that have a low glycemic index, such as apples, berries, peaches, pears, plums, oranges, and grapefruit. On the other hand, dates and raisins are high in sugar.

- Nuts, such as walnuts and almonds, are good snacks—but only eat about 15 of any type of nut at any given time because of the many calories that nuts contain.

- Celery sticks and baby carrots are also good snacks. Carrots have a low glycemic load and are very high in fiber, which slows down the absorption of sugar and lowers blood sugar.

- Granola is incredibly high on the glycemic index, but you can substitute granola with a high-fiber cereal, a protein smoothie, an egg-white omelet, or some steel-cut oats.

- If you are trying to lower your blood sugar, you need to find healthier alternatives for cookies, cakes, candy, and ice cream. In addition, you should not drink soda, fruit juice, or alcohol. You also need to find substitutes for anything white—whether it's a bagel, bread, rice cakes, or potatoes.

- You can also use spices in a creative way. For example, add cinnamon—which has been shown to lower blood sugar—and a few walnuts to steel-cut oats for breakfast. Instead of drinking coffee with cream in it, start drinking organic green tea.

- Garlic and onions help bring down blood sugar. You should focus on eating green leafy vegetables with light amounts of olive oil and turmeric, an anti-inflammatory, on top.

- Fenugreek comes out of Ayurvedic medicine from India and can be used as a spice that lowers blood sugar. There are also properties in vinegar that have been shown to lower blood sugar.

Preventing and Reversing Diabetes: Physical Activity
- On average, Americans spend six hours per day in front of a television or computer, so make sure that you are making time for exercise—which builds muscle, decreases insulin resistance, decreases blood pressure, improves cholesterol, and improves your sense of well-being.

- Make a commitment with a friend to start exercising together, and hold each other responsible for your exercise. You can also attend a dance class, such as a Nia class, which is a combination of dance and Tai Chi.

- One of the best added benefits of exercise is that it helps you sleep better. Use a pedometer, a small device that counts the number of steps that you take, and work toward the goal of taking 10,000 steps each day.

1. What is the glycemic index?

2. Name three lifestyle changes that can impact insulin resistance, metabolic syndrome, and diabetes.

Treating Diabetes Naturally
Lecture 12—Transcript

Welcome back. Today we get to talk about one of my favorite topics. We will talk about a spectrum of sugar (metabolism) disorders that range on one end from pre-diabetes to full blown diabetes. Now, I'm not going to talk about the kind of diabetes that happens early in life. That is the type of diabetes when the pancreas fails for some reason and stops making insulin. This is when we see young people requiring insulin injections. I'm going to be talking about the kind of diabetes that results from lifestyle; what kind of food we eat, how physically active we are, and how we respond to stress and tension. In short how we live our lives.

So why is diabetes so important? We've already heard about the importance of high cholesterol and high blood pressure. Well diabetes is one of the key risk factors for kidney disease leading to dialysis, heart disease, and stroke. In fact if I see a woman coming into my office after having a heart attack the first question I think about is, "Is she smoking cigarettes or is she diabetic?" That's how big a risk factor it is. Diabetes affects every single organ in our body.

We need to think of the diagnosis of diabetes as the end result of a much longer continuum. The continuum starts with something called insulin resistance and then metabolic syndrome before manifesting the disease that we label as diabetes. This is important because in other words even before the blood tests tell us that you have diabetes we have signs that can be seen much earlier. Let's look at this spectrum and review a few of these definitions.

One of the first signs that we are at risk for developing diabetes is the presence of insulin resistance. Insulin is a hormone which controls blood sugar. Insulin is produced by the pancreas. Stimuli like insulin and even exercise carry blood sugar into our cell so we need the insulin to move the sugar into our cells where we can use it for energy. Insulin resistance occurs when the transport of sugar into the cell is no longer working properly. The pancreas has to keep working harder and harder to produce more insulin. High insulin levels on a blood test will tell us if you have insulin resistance.

Eventually, the pancreas can't keep up; it gets exhausted and can't produce enough insulin. That's when people develop insulin requiring diabetes and those people need insulin injections.

But the story does not stop there. Insulin resistance is part of a larger syndrome called metabolic syndrome. Metabolic syndrome has four components. Number one is insulin resistance. Number two is high blood pressure. Number three is abnormalities in the cholesterol panel. That means the HDL or good cholesterol could be low and the triglycerides are high. Remember the seesaw, triglycerides are up, HDL is down. These are the first three components of the metabolic syndrome. The forth component of metabolic syndrome is really what's driving the train toward diabetes and that is abdominal obesity; wearing your weight in the midline. Yes that's right, extra weight in the midline will cause diabetes and a lot of other problems as well. Extra midline weight is linked to heart disease, believe it or not to osteoporosis, even Alzheimer's disease, high blood pressure, and high cholesterol—and these are just a few.

The Center for Disease Control tells us that obesity is a "Major Public Health Threat." Nearly 27 percent of adults in the United States are now obese. That's 72 million Americans. The health-care implications of obesity are enormous. By the end of the decade, it is predicted that the annual cost for diabetes and pre-diabetes alone will be $500 billion.

Let's say you have that diagnosis of diabetes or you have metabolic syndrome or you have already evidence of insulin resistance, you have high insulin levels in your blood and you go to your physician. Well you physician is going to name that disease. Remember we discussed this in the first couple of lectures. Your physician is going to name the disease and is going to prescribe a medication. The ill to the pill; this is the classic way metabolic syndrome, diabetes, and insulin resistance are handled. Now think about this for a few seconds. I already said that metabolic syndrome has high blood pressure associated with it, cholesterol abnormalities, blood sugar abnormalities, central obesity, guess how many pills you're going to get. You're going to get a pill for insulin resistance, you're going to get a pill for high blood pressure, you're going to get a pill for cholesterol and your physician is going to say you need to take an aspirin too because, rightfully so, you are at an increased risk for heart disease.

But now you've been listening to this course and because you are listening to the Science of Natural Healing you now know, even if you take those medications you have to ask the question, "What's going on in my soil? What's happening to make me sick that leads to all of these diagnoses? Why is the fruit on my tree sick?"

Well I have a great patient named Ron. He came to me after having bypass surgery and he'll be thrilled to know that I'm talking about him in this course. Diabetes was his biggest risk factor for heart disease. Ron was 168 pounds overweight. By the time he came to me, he said, "I need to get off the tracks. I want to get to the underlying cause of my problems. I want to get this diabetes fixed." In essence what Ron was saying is, "Help me to strengthen my soil." So I told Ron there are five key steps that he needs to take to strengthen his soil. And at the time he came to see me, he was ready to hear them. I told him that we need to look at 1) what he's eating, proper nutrition; 2) Is he exercising every day? What is his physical activity? 3) Is he a hothead? How does he respond to stress and tension? 4) Is he sleeping well at night? And 5) I told Ron that even environmental toxins can make his diabetes worse.

Let's take number four, for example. Most people don't realize lack of sleep can lead to insulin resistance. Lack of sleep is a stress on the body and as you will hear in later lectures, stress raises blood sugar and makes insulin resistance worse. Well Ron had something we see in people that are very overweight. He had something called sleep apnea. This is when you go to sleep at night and you snore and you stop breathing. This was a result of being obese. Research shows that people who tend to clock an average of five hours or less of sleep each night have a higher risk of developing diabetes.

As for stress and environmental toxins, these areas are so important that they will be covered in separate lectures. For Ron, the best place to start was nutrition and exercise. So let's look at some of these areas and let's make some literally life saving recommendations for Ron.

Let's start with my favorite topic, nutrition. Remember food is medicine. Now sugar and carbohydrates are digested at different rates. The rate of digestion is called the glycemic index. The higher the index the faster the body converts that food to sugar. Let me give you an example. A spoonful of white sugar has a glycemic index of 100. That's the highest number a food can have. The minute you eat that white sugar it goes right into your bloodstream within seconds. Another way of measuring the conversion of food to sugar is called the glycemic load. Now this is a little bit more complicated because the glycemic load is an even more accurate assessment of the impact of food on blood sugar and ultimately on insulin levels.

A food with a glycemic load of greater than 20 is high. A food with a glycemic load of less than 10 is low. For me, when it comes to glycemic index and glycemic load, the lowest possible foods are the best for everyone, but especially for someone who's overweight or pre-diabetic or has diabetes. Let's look at the difference. Let's take a carrot, perfect example. The glycemic index of a carrot is 16, but the glycemic load is two, so carrots are okay. Why is the glycemic load less than the glycemic index? Because in this case carrots are very high in fiber. When we eat a food that's high in fiber, and you've heard this before, it slows down the absorption of sugar. Fiber, as you already know, will also lower blood sugar so that makes carrots a good choice with a low glycemic load.

So how do I want Ron to eat and ultimately how do I eat and how do I want you to eat? The most important thing I can teach you about food as it relates to inflammation and health is that I don't want you to eat foods that spike up your insulin level. Insulin has been linked to cancers, it leads as we have discussed to inflammation, and every time we spike up our insulin we are making ourselves sick. Foods that have a low glycemic index and a low glycemic load are the foods that I want Ron and I want you to eat.

We already discussed many of these foods, and I know you're going to say, "I know, I know," but I'll say it again: Soluble fiber lowers cholesterol, lowers blood sugar—oats and bran, beans and lentils. Let's get our green leafy vegetables onboard. Green leafy vegetables have a very, very low glycemic load and low glycemic index. Cruciferous vegetables like cauliflower, broccoli, and cabbage are all good choices. Omega-3 fish, remember we have salmon, we have mackerel, we have anchovy, we have sardines, and we have herring (you remember the word SMASH), and Omega-3 eggs. If you're going to eat meat, lean meat like free range chicken and turkey, these will not spike up your insulin.

I told Ron I wanted him to pick his fruits from a low glycemic index list. What does that mean? I literally handed him a handout that said eat this and don't eat that. I told him he can eat three whole fruits a day, but they had to be low sugar fruits: apples, berries, peaches, pears, plums. He can have an orange, but not orange juice, right. He can have a grapefruit. These are all low in sugar. One thing I had to tell him that he was eating a lot of was dates and raisins and I said, "Ron, dates and raisins are too high in sugar."

What about for snacks? he said. I recommended some walnuts, some almonds—and remember the magic number around 15. Ron has 168 pounds to decrease so I don't want him having too many calories from nuts. I also suggested celery sticks, baby carrots, and I even told Ron to take an apple or take a pear and put it in a pot with some water and soften it up, make a warm apple. And if he wants I told him to put cinnamon on it because cinnamon has been shown to lower blood sugar.

He was very concerned with what he can eat in the morning. What kind of breakfast cereal can he have? He was already eating granola and I had to point out that granola is incredibly high on the glycemic index so we needed a substitute. I had him pick a high fiber cereal and on some mornings I asked him to make a protein smoothie and maybe to make an egg white omelet and also to use steel cut oats so he had lots of choices.

The hard part for Ron is I had to tell him to stop certain foods. I don't like to focus on what we can't eat because years ago my patients used to call me Dr. No. When I was a young physician I used to say no don't eat that, no don't eat this and I realized that's not the way to do it. Foods like cookies, cakes, candy, and ice cream, I had to tell Ron we have to start substituting our baked apple and baked pear. I had to remind him about the liquid calories and I will say no soda, no fruit juice, and small to none on the alcohol. Alcohol is calories and it's sugar, and it wouldn't serve him well in this situation. I also had to tell Ron to resist the white stuff. If it's white, whether it's a bagel, bread, even whole wheat, rice cakes, potatoes, I had to tell him we need to find substitutes for all these foods.

Now one area that was confusing Ron, that confuses a lot of my patients, is in label reading. When you look at the labels if you see the words corn syrup, high fructose corn syrup, dextrose, fructose, maltose, and sucrose, those are all other names for sugar. It's sugar hidden by another name. If you need to get your sugar down, get your weight off, you don't want to be eating it. By the way, if you can't read a label on a box, if it sounds like a chemistry experiment, why would we be eating that food anyway?

Let's take a look at what else we can do. I've already taught Ron that I wanted him to use spices, for example, in a creative way. After I mentioned cinnamon, he told me he really likes it so I said let's add cinnamon to the steel cut oats in the morning and I also told him to add a couple of halves of walnuts to his steel cut oats. If he wanted a serving of fruit in the morning I recommended adding some blueberries or berries of any type and I also recommended that he not add any coffee and cream to his regimen. You might say what's better. I asked Ron to start drinking organic green tea so we were able to come up with some creative ways to start building good spices into his food.

I told him that I wanted him to use garlic and onions as much as he liked. Garlic and onions actually help to bring down blood sugar so all the green leafy vegetables he wants with light amounts of olive oil, garlic as we've talked about in the past and then I even recommended that he use turmeric on top. Why did I recommend turmeric? Because it's anti-inflammatory; when you are diabetic, you are inflamed. Your heart is on fire so we want to cool that fire down.

What else can he do? I recommended something fenugreek. Now this comes out of Ayurveda medicine from India and it can be used as a spice and it's very common in Indian cuisine. I also recommended that he use vinegar because there're actually properties in vinegar, if he likes it on his salad, that have been shown to lower blood s2gar. We spent a lot of time going over nutrition because nutrition is key to shifting the diabetes continuum. We can't fix the problem if we keep eating white bread and white rice and white pasta. It just won't work.

So what's next. Ron now knows how to eat. Well at Great Courses they have a sign that says Bottoms UP. I like this sign. I find it kind of funny. They don't mean lets go to the bar and have a drink. They mean get your butt off the chair and start to move. Do you know on average Americans are spending six hours in front of a TV set or in front of a computer. Well if you want to be at your computer for six hours than I suggest you stand up. Better yet, you can get one of those new desks that actually has a treadmill built in it so you can do your work and be on the treadmill at the same time. Simple exercise like walking burns calories. Exercise builds muscle. Exercise decreases insulin resistance. The cell becomes more sensitive to the insulin and the sugar can move in easier. Exercise decreases blood pressure. It improves cholesterol and it absolutely improves our sense of well-being.

Now this is one of the jokes I tell my patients. If you won't exercise on your own you have to get a friend who's willing to exercise with you. I always tell the ladies get a good looking personal trainer; that will get you to the gym. Make a commitment with a friend to start to exercise.

You know I have a treadmill in my garage. What's more boring than that? Walking on a treadmill in your garage, no fun at all. I don't look forward to it. I look forward to taking my dog, my poodle Sam, and walking with me and he looks forward to it almost as much as I do. Get a friend, get a partner, hold each other responsible for your exercise and there'll be many days when you'll say I don't feel like going and your friend will say oh come we're going. There'll be other days when you'll tell your friend hey let's get going. Another fun thing to do is go to a dance class. My heart patients love our dance classes. You know, I forgot that in the 1940s and '50s that people used to go out every night almost and dance, ballroom dancing. I walked into a Nia class, which is a combination of dance and Tai Chi and my patients were having a ball. They loved it. They were exercising and they were smiling. That's a great combination.

And one of the biggest added benefits of exercise is it helps us to get a good night's sleep. When someone says to me I have insomnia, I'm watching the clock all night, the first thing I ask is do you exercise. It's that important. So where do we start? When someone leaves my office, I give them a little pedometer, a little device to count the number of steps that they take. You can buy a pedometer almost anywhere. They are cheap; they're easy to find. I just give them away because I like when my patients leave I like to see it on their belt. Your goal is 10,000 steps each day! You may not be ready to start at 10,000 steps, you might say, "Dr. G. you're crazy; I don't even do five steps!" Just get up and get started and everyday you increase it by a few steps. You may not get there on the first day, but I guarantee it you will definitely get there if you keep going.

Now you have the tools that can prevent and even reverse diabetes. Go ahead make a commitment. Go clean out that pantry and refrigerator and fill them with good whole foods. Get rid of the high fructose corn syrup, the trans fats, the partially hydrogenated oils, the white stuff; clean it all out. Go and buy a pedometer and take that first big step! Remember this: You can't get anywhere if you don't start somewhere!

Stress and the Mind-Body Connection
Lecture 13

In this lecture, you will learn about the stress response and the three key stress hormones, which are adrenaline, aldosterone, and cortisol. You will also learn that there are 1,400 chemical reactions that occur when you are under stress. In addition, you will discover some compelling research that addresses how stress can affect your health. Some of this research clearly demonstrates that stress—both acute stress and chronic stress—will make you sick.

The Pervasive Nature of Stress

- The American Institute of Stress reports that 75 to 90 percent of all visits to health-care providers result from stress-related disorders.

- Stress is a state one experiences when there is a mismatch between perceived demands and our ability to cope. In other words, stress is experienced when people don't feel like they can do everything that is expected of them.

- Stress has been extensively studied in the military, and a very insightful model of stress was developed during World War II to understand what happens to soldiers when they are on the battlefield, exposed to hundreds—if not thousands—of stressful situations. For some of us, our work or home environment can sometimes feel like a war zone, and our ability to perform at our best can be seriously impacted in similar ways.

- People who think that stress is good are typically confusing stress with challenge. At first, challenge improves our performance, but as the amount of work continues and our challenges in life increase, our ability to perform our best can be compromised.

Stress and the Body

- When under stress, the body goes through several physiological changes that can be measured and quantified, including an increase in heart rate, blood sugar, breathing rate, and blood pressure.

- The autonomic, or automatic, nervous system has two components: the sympathetic nervous system, which is the stimulating nervous system, and the parasympathetic nervous system, which is the system that makes you calm and relaxed.

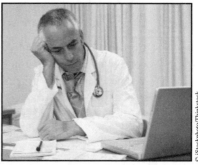

- When your sympathetic nervous system is activated, your blood becomes stickier and more prone to clot. You also produce hormones—a few of which raise your blood pressure, such as renin and angiotensin. In addition, your insulin resistance increases, so your fasting insulin increases. Furthermore, cholesterol and blood pressure rise, and arteries constrict.

Physicians are aware that stress has negative emotional, mental, and physical effects on the human body.

- There are over 1,400 chemical reactions that occur in our bodies as a result of stress. There are three key stress hormones that support our bodies in emergency situations: adrenaline, aldosterone, and cortisol.

- Adrenaline is a hormone that is produced by the adrenal gland, which sits on top of the kidneys. Adrenaline is produced during high-stress or exciting situations and is part of your body's acute stress response—called the fight-or-flight reaction.

- When you produce adrenaline, your heart rate increases, your blood vessels constrict, and your airways dilate—all of which bring more blood flow to your muscles and more oxygen to your lungs.

- Aldosterone is essential to life because it regulates electrolytes, which include elements such as sodium and potassium. Aldosterone is also secreted by the adrenal gland and causes the reabsorption of sodium, which is needed in stressful situations, into the bloodstream.

- Cortisol is also produced by the adrenal gland, and you need cortisol to release sugar into your bloodstream under stress because you need sugar in your muscles when they are being used.

- Cortisol is associated with another hormone called DHEA, which can be thought of as the happy hormone. When cortisol increases, DHEA decreases.

- These three hormones play an important role in our survival. The key is that they are triggered in emergency situations, which arise quickly and hopefully subside just as quickly.

- However, if we never turn our stress hormones off, our blood pressure increases, and we end up with ulcers in our stomach and are more prone to infections and even cancer. The male hormone testosterone decreases, and women have irregular menstrual cycles.

Emotional and Mental Effects of Stress

- Stress not only causes physical changes in our bodies, but it also causes emotional and mental changes. Research shows that people under stress have cognitive inhibition, causing them to not make the best choices. Stress causes us to lose focus; it affects our mental clarity.

- Stress affects our ability to relax and sleep, and when we feel as though we cannot cope with all of the items on our agenda, stress even affects our self-esteem.

- Stress also leads to anger, which increases the risk of a heart attack by 230 percent. Anger is one of the most lethal emotions for the heart.

- There has been a lot of research on the impact of stress in both acute and chronic situations. Research that assessed heart patients one month after the terrorist attacks of September 11, 2001, showed that there was a 2.3-fold increase in ventricular tachyarrhythmias, which are the bad arrhythmias that cause sudden death.

- Research by Dr. Janice Kiecolt-Glaser in the area of chronic stress shows that caregiving is a good thing, but if you deplete yourself and make yourself physically, emotionally, and mentally exhausted as a result of giving care to another, it will affect your immune system.

- Dr. Kiecolt-Glaser's work shows that if a physician administers the flu vaccine to caregivers who are depleted and exhausted, they may not even mount the response to the flu vaccine— meaning that they do not get the antibodies to protect them. Perhaps they were under so much stress that they could not produce antibodies.

- Chronic stress is an interesting area of research. High cortisol levels and low DHEA levels are associated with accelerated aging, impaired memory and ability to learn, and even osteoporosis. In other words, chronic stress will cause bone loss. There is another sign of aging that comes with chronic stress: a reduction in muscle mass.

- Under stress, immune function is affected and blood sugar increases. Stress also makes diabetes much worse. Furthermore, high levels of cortisol makes people gain weight.

1. Name three stress hormones.

2. Name one mental condition and two physical conditions that are caused by stress.

Stress and the Mind-Body Connection
Lecture 13—Transcript

When I went to medical school I did not have one single lecture on how stress can affect health. Yet, when I ask my patients if they are under stress the answer is almost always yes! Today we will discuss the stress response, the stress hormones, and some compelling research on how stress can make us sick. The former U.S. Surgeon General, Julius Richmond, had this to say, "Of the ten leading causes of illness and death in the United States, seven could be greatly reduced if the following lifestyle habits were modified— alcohol abuse, lack of exercise, poor diet, smoking, and unhealthy … responses to stress and tension."

We have in this country something called the American Institute of Stress. And one of their staggering statistics is that 75 to 90 percent of all visits to health care providers result from stress-related disorders. Now when I first saw this number, I thought this is way too high. It's not possible; 75 to 90 percent of all visits are related to stress. I started to keep a little checklist of why people were coming to see me. Things like chest pain, patients would come with high blood pressure. They would come with diabetes. They would come with irritable bowel syndrome, muscle spasms, and headaches. All of these are related to stress. I finally gave in and I realized that the American Institute of Stress was right all along, 75 to 90 percent of all visits to health-care providers are related to stress.

What is stress? How would we define it? I like this definition. "Stress can be defined as a state one experiences when there is a mismatch between perceived demands and our ability to cope." What does that mean? I have so many things to do I can't get to all of them. I don't feel like I can do everything that is expected of me. When we feel like we can't cope, that's when we're stressed. If we feel like we can get the job done, we usually do it with a smile.

Stress has been extensively studied in the military and a very insightful model of stress was developed during World War II to understand what happens to soldiers when they are on the battlefield exposed to hundreds, if not thousands, of stressful situations. Now for some of us, our work or our home environment can sometimes feel like a war zone. I have actually heard people use this description to describe their home, and our ability to perform at our best can be seriously impacted in much the same way. People who think stress is good usually don't mean stress. They mean challenge. Challenge at first improves our performance. I have to do a series of lectures today; that's a challenge, but I'm looking forward to it. I don't see it as a stress. But as the amount of work continues and our challenges in life increase, our ability to perform our best can be compromised.

I see this with my young physicians all the time when they come out of medical school they are so happy to have a pager. At my age I'm happy to give that thing away. They come out and they are great on the wards in the hospital, treating patients and doing everything 100 percent, but then sometimes life gets in the way, even good things. What I see happen with my young physicians is when they first come out of medical school they don't have all the demands on them of family and spouse and owning a house. They haven't even paid back their student loans so their plate just has on it "treat the patients." One thing: keep the patients healthy. Now they get married, they have kids, they keep piling things onto their plate and this is when they come to me and they say, "I'm feeling burned out." They no longer can cope. So the amount of work or challenge becomes more and more and the ability to perform is compromised.

What do we typically do in a situation like this? We decide, "I just have to work longer. I'm going to put in more hours. I'm going to work harder just to keep up." Most people don't notice, but performance begins to slip. We are just not doing things as well as we used to. Left unchecked like those medical students, you and I will eventually become exhausted, wiped out, and maybe even burned out.

What happens to the body when we are under stress? When under stress we see a lot of physiologic changes, changes in the body that actually can be measured and quantified. Let's start with the most obvious one, an increase in heart rate. Now not everyone likes to give public lectures. If I told you today was your day to give a public lecture you might get nervous if you don't like to do that. The first thing you would notice is your heart would start to pound. You would notice an increase in your heart rate. Stress does other things as well. It increases your blood sugar. It increases your breathing rate. It increases your blood pressure, and the list is endless.

Let's take a minute here to talk about the autonomic nervous system. Autonomic means automatic, things that the body will do without you telling it. What's an example? You go to sleep at night and you breathe. You breathe throughout the night. You don't have to tell your body to take a breath, take a breath, it happens automatically. The autonomic nervous system has two components. I like to think of these as a seesaw. On one end we have the sympathetic nervous system; that is the stimulating nervous system. That is the one that gets me up and going. On the other end, we have the parasympathetic nervous system. That's the one that makes me calm and relaxed. Think about it this way. Sympathetic nervous system: My foot is on the gas. Parasympathetic nervous system: My foot is on the brake.

What happens when our sympathetic nervous system is up and going? What happens in our body if our foot is on the gas all the time? Well the first thing we see is changes in our blood. Our blood becomes stickier, more prone to clot. We also produce hormones. A few raise your blood pressure. Renin and angiotensin cause the blood pressure to go up. Our insulin resistance increases so our fasting insulin, which we talked about, goes up. Even cholesterol goes up, blood pressure goes up, and arteries constrict.

Many years ago, I thought about this list and I thought about the medications that I am giving everyday to my heart patients. Let's take a look quickly. I give aspirin and Plavix as blood thinners. Well that is blocking the coagulation problem. I give blood pressure medicines, well that blocks that renin and angiotensin problem that I mentioned. Then I might give cholesterol medicine, which is going to block the effect of high cholesterol, and so on. The take home message for me was yes your medicines are good, but maybe what I need to be doing with my patients is medicate and also, as you'll see, meditate.

We have over 1400 chemical reactions in our body that occur as a result of stress. For the purpose of this lecture we will talk about three key stress hormones, adrenaline, aldosterone, and the third stress hormone is cortisol. Let's take a look at these three. Let's start with adrenaline.

Adrenaline is a hormone produced by the adrenal gland. The adrenal gland looks like a little hat. It sits on top of our kidneys. Adrenaline is produced during high stress or exciting situations. You can produce adrenaline even in a happy situation. This hormone is part of our body's acute stress response (you have all heard this before): the "fight or flight" reaction. When we produce adrenaline our heart rate goes up. Our blood vessels constrict, even our air ways dilate, all of which brings more blood flow to our muscles and more oxygen to our lungs. Why would this occur in a fight or flight reaction? Think about that for a second.

A tiger is chasing us. Do I need an increased heart rate? Absolutely, because I need to get blood to my muscles because you can bet I'm running. I'm not even fighting; I'm running. The hormone is there to help us out.

Aldosterone, the second stress hormone, is also there to help us out. This hormone is absolutely essential to life because it regulates our electrolytes. Our electrolytes are things like sodium and potassium for example. Aldosterone is also secreted by the adrenal gland and it causes the re-absorption of sodium into the bloodstream. Now you may be thinking, "Dr. G. told me sodium is bad, why would I want more of that in my bloodstream? It's going to raise my blood pressure. I listened to that lecture." Well that's true. But, think about it in the setting of acute stress.

Let's say someone has an automobile accident and they are bleeding to death. The stress hormones kick in to save that person's life. Because they are bleeding, their blood pressure is going down so aldosterone is pulling back all the sodium to raise the blood pressure while adrenaline is constricting the blood vessels to stop the bleeding. These hormones are crucial for our lifesaving situations.

Let's take a look at the third, cortisol. Cortisol is a little bit different. It is also produced by the adrenal gland and I used to always think cortisol was bad, but cortisol is not bad. We need cortisol to release sugar into our bloodstream. Why under stress do we need sugar? We need sugar because remember we are running or we are fighting so we need sugar in our muscles. Taken together cortisol, adrenaline, and aldosterone are there to support us in emergency situations.

We have another seesaw here that I need to mention. Cortisol keeps company with another hormone called DHEA. Now DHEA, remember the H there stands for happy. This is our happy hormone. And please don't go out and start taking DHEA tablets because I'm going to teach you how to lower your cortisol and raise your DHEA naturally, but for the purposes of this lecture when cortisol goes up our happy hormone, DHEA, goes down.

So these hormones all play an important role in our survival. The key is that this function is triggered in emergency situations, situations that come quickly and hopefully go away as quickly. These hormones are not there for us as a way of life. But what happens if we never turn the stress hormones off? What happens if we constantly release these hormones into our bloodstream? If we never turn our stress hormones off our blood pressure goes up, we end up with ulcers in our stomach. Our hormonal system gets affected. In men, the male hormone testosterone goes down. Women get irregular menstrual cycles and we are more prone to infections and even cancer.

But the story does not end there. Stress does not only cause physical changes in our body, stress also causes emotional and mental changes. I bet many of you already know what these are. I don't know about you, but if I'm under stress, I find that I am not thinking clearly. The research shows that people under stress have something called cognitive inhibition, the ability to use the brain that God gave us. We don't make the best choices under stress. A perfect example, if you are feeling stressed have you ever said something you regretted five seconds later. I think we all have. Stress causes us to lose our focus; it affects our mental clarity. Everyone knows it affects the ability to relax and to sleep and when we have a lot of things on our plate and we feel like we can't cope, it even affects our self esteem, we will absolutely feel exhausted and I can't tell you how many huge cardiac workups I have done on patients when they come in and they say to me I feel tired and that is their main complaint. Of course, I want to make sure is it their heart, is it their thyroid, are they anemic. What's going on? Many times at the end of the day I find out it is stress.

The other thing we see is anger. Let's take a look at some of the research on the impact of stress in both acute and chronic situations. Let's take a look at what's in the medical literature. We'll start with one of my favorites from the

British Medical Journal in 2002. There was a 25 percent increase in heart attack admissions in London on the day of the match when England lost to Argentina in a penalty shootout during the 1998 World Cup. Think about that for a second. You have seen your friends during a Super Bowl game or during the World Series. Those are the stress hormones in action. I remember when I was a young resident at Cornell and I used to work in the emergency room and I told my chief resident one day, "I'll work any night of the week but Monday night," and he asked me why. I said. "Because all these guys are coming in with chest pain and heart failure, congestive heart failure, all sorts of things are going on on Monday night." I never connected it to Monday Night Football until I started to understand the impact of stress.

We had a large earthquake in California in the 1990s; it was called the Northridge earthquake. The LA County Coroner reported five times higher increase in cardiovascular disease-related sudden deaths on the day of the Northridge earthquake. That means people dying suddenly of things related to the heart; this is not a car accident, on the day of the earthquake. Again, the concept of acute stress having very devastating consequences. I don't know about you, but I can tell you exactly where I was on 9/11. I think most of us remember that day and have it etched in our hearts forever. What the research showed if we looked at heart patients one month after 9/11, there was a 2.3-fold increase in ventricular tachyarrhythmias. These are the bad arrhythmias, the ones that cause sudden death, and it lasted for one month after 9/11.

Now I mentioned anger as something that frequently happens when we are under stress. You know when people ask you one more thing or ask one more thing of you and you feel like you have nothing left to give. We the research on anger is really clear. Anger increases the risk of a heart attack 230 percent. Think of how we describe angry people. We say, "Oh they're a hothead, oh their blood is boiling." Well their blood is boiling because their platelets are sticky and yes they are a hothead and they turn red because their blood pressure is so high. So anger is one of the most lethal emotions for the heart. What I tell my patients is this. You may not think you are the angry person, but I suggest you ask your spouse or you ask your employees and they will let you know if you're the angry person because this is one of those areas where the people don't like to admit that about themselves.

Let's take a look at some of the research on chronic stress. Louis Pasteur said this, "The microbe is nothing, the soil is everything." Isn't that the essence of our entire seminar? The soil is everything. Now if I was to take the rhinovirus, the virus that causes colds, and I was to pump it in a room filled with people would everyone get the rhinovirus? I know you're saying no. Well what determines who gets the rhinovirus and who doesn't? What determines it is our resiliency, how good our soil is, our micronutrition, our macronutrition, the way we respond to stress and to tension. This is what determines it, how much we sleep and so on. So let's look at some of the research in this area.

Dr. Glazer is an amazing researcher. She has done more in the area of understanding chronic stress than anyone that I know. One of her first studies was to look at what happens if we do a simple punch biopsy, just take a little piece of skin from caregivers and from very good well-matched controls, people who are not caregivers. It took caregivers, on average, 24 percent longer to heal the same wound. The way I teach it to my patients is this way, when you go on the airplane and they tell you if the oxygen mask falls what do they say? Do they say put it on the guy next to you? No. They say to put it on yourself first then you can help others. Well this is the oxygen mask analogy. Caregiving is a good thing, but if you deplete yourself and make yourself physically, emotionally, mentally exhausted it will affect your immune system.

Dr. Glazer did a second study, this time looking at medical students. She said what if we do that same simple punch biopsy in medical students during exam week and while they are on vacation. What she found was that it took the medical students, on average, 40 percent longer to heal this simple wound during their exam week. Why? Because they were under stress and their immune system, their ability to heal wounds and to fight, was affected.

In the fall I give many of my patients, especially those that would like it, the flu vaccine. I never really thought about who I was giving the flu vaccine to, we offered it to everyone. Again, Dr. Glazer's work shows that if you give the flu vaccine to a caregiver who is depleted and exhausted they may not even mount the response to the flu vaccine meaning they do not get the antibodies to protect them. Maybe that's why so many people come in and say wow I had the flu vaccine and I got the flu and we almost always say, "Oh it was a different strain." That may be true, but maybe they were under so much stress that they could not even produce the antibodies to protect them.

Well this is an interesting area of research because if we look at that seesaw again, high cortisol, low DHEA, let's take a look at what the research shows us. The first and obvious one is accelerated aging. I hate to say it, but take a look at any U.S. president when they come into office and when they leave office. That is a perfect example of accelerated aging. We know that high cortisol and low DHEA impair our memory and our ability to learn. What most people do not realize is it also causes osteoporosis. People talk all the time about their bones and they say, "I have to get more calcium, more magnesium, more vitamin D," and yes that's all very important, but you also have to factor in stress. If you are under chronic stress it will cause bone loss.

There is another sign of aging that comes with chronic stress. We lose our muscle. We have a reduction in our muscle mass. We already mentioned our immune function is affected under stress. Remember those students who couldn't heal the simple little punch biopsy. Our blood sugar goes up, stress will make diabetes much worse, and last but not least, cortisol will make us fat. It puts weight on in our midline and weight in our hips, so just being under stress can put pounds on you. There's something else that we do when we're under stress that leads to weight gain: We tend to eat mindlessly. I know in my family, the Italians, if there is a crisis in the house everyone goes to the kitchen. My aunt starts cooking and everyone starts eating. That is how we cope. That is how we were raised to cope so just having high cortisol will put weight on in your midline.

Today we have learned a lot about the stress response. We discussed the three stress hormones adrenaline, aldosterone, and cortisol and remember we said there are 1400 chemical reactions that occur when we are under stress. We have seen research that clearly demonstrates that stress will make us sick, both acute stress and chronic stress, unless we figure out a way to turn stress into strength. And that is the subject of our next lecture.

Turning Stress into Strength
Lecture 14

In this lecture, you will be introduced to biological interventions that can help you turn stress into strength. Stress is almost always an emotional reaction to a situation, and it impacts your ability to think clearly, respond appropriately, and perform at your best. Your stress level impacts not only how you feel at the end of the day, but it also impacts your health and even your relationships. This lecture focuses on the power of positive emotions, and you will learn a powerful technique to neutralize stress called heart-focused breathing.

The Effects of Perception

- Frequently, you can't control the world around you. It is the initiating events that occur that we cannot control, but we can control our perception of those events—which leads to the physical response that involves releasing the stress hormones.

- Stress is not the situation; it is your mental and emotional reactions to the situation.

- In a research study on how people's perceptions of the world affect their health, students were asked to watch a movie about Mother Teresa's activities, including administering to the sick and taking care of the poor. A protein that protects the body from infection, called IgA, was measured.

- In about 92 percent of the students, IgA levels increased after watching the movie about Mother Teresa. In other words, their immune systems were positively affected. However, in about eight percent of the students, IgA levels decreased after watching the movie.

- The students were then asked to write a story about a picture of a couple on a park bench. All they could see from the picture was the backs of a man and a woman sitting on a park bench.

- The students whose IgA levels had increased came up with stories about proposals and marriage. However, the other eight percent, whose immune system had decreased after watching the Mother Teresa movie, came up with stories about distrust, manipulation, and abandonment. In other words, these students saw everything negatively. They even claimed to dislike Mother Teresa.

- When the researchers looked at who were the sickest students over the previous year, it was those students who had the negative response to the Mother Teresa movie that were sick all the time. The researchers concluded that perception was the key.

Reacting to Stress

- We may not be able to change various aspects of our environment, but we can change how we react to, and perceive, our environment.

- If you find yourself experiencing negative thoughts and having negative emotions, it is important to know how to shift your thoughts, thereby shifting the consequences of the stress hormones.

- Research has shown that people who generally have positive thoughts—the optimists of the world—have increased longevity.

- Positive emotions reduce morbidity from various diseases, and they result in us having more cognitive flexibility—more creativity. Having positive emotions cause us to be better at problem solving and more innovative. Positive emotions even improve our job performance.

- Not just thinking about a positive emotion, but actually feeling a positive emotion is what has a positive effect on your body.

- People who see the world negatively should try keeping a gratefulness journal. At night, they should write down things that they are grateful for so that they start feeling love and getting the physiologic benefits from having positive emotions.

- When you are in a stressful situation or are thinking negative thoughts, start by neutralizing the negative thoughts and feelings. Take a time-out—which involves sitting down and taking a few deep breaths—before you say something or do something that you are going to regret.

Heart-Focused Breathing

- Breathing controls our autonomic nervous system. When we take a deep breath in, our heart rate increases, and when we exhale, our heart rate decreases. However, if we breathe in a cyclical, rhythmical way, it stabilizes our autonomic nervous system.

- To engage in heart-focused breathing, the first thing you need to do is to take a time-out. Remove yourself from the stressful situation.

- Most of us breathe from the upper third of our lungs. Take a deep breath—what is called a yogic breath in yoga terms—for five seconds in and five seconds out. As soon as you start the breath, it interrupts the body's stress response, so you should already start to feel more relaxed.

- Next, draw your focus down to your heart; imagine that you are breathing in and out through your heart. This may feel strange at first, but in a few minutes, it will become more natural. This is called heart breathing. Keep breathing for five seconds in and five seconds out.

- If you are having trouble doing this for the first time, you may want to place your right hand over your heart, and if it is comfortable, place your left hand over your right hand, and begin to breathe in and out.

- You may also find that closing your eyes will make this breathing technique easier. With practice, you will be able to do it with your eyes opened or closed.

- If you have a problem that you are trying to solve but cannot get the solution, engage in some heart-focused breathing, but also think about something that elicits a positive emotion for you while you are breathing. Don't just think about unconditional love or appreciation; actually feel the gratefulness.

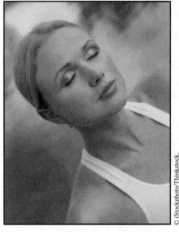

- Adding the power of positive emotion can improve your cognition, increase your mental flexibility, and help you make decisions. One of the easiest ways to do this is to remember a special place or someone you love or appreciate.

If you are feeling stressed, simply close your eyes and breathe in for five seconds and out for five seconds.

- After adding the power of positive emotion—by thinking about your child, grandchild, or puppy, for example—hold that feeling of appreciation or love for about 20 seconds. Then, radiate that love to yourself and to all those around you.

- When you catch your mind wandering away and find that you cannot retain your focus, do not be upset. Instead, always return your focus to the breathing. Then, reconnect with your feelings of caring, love, and appreciation.

- If you have a problem that you have not been able to solve with your mind, your heart might be able to solve it for you if you engage in heart-focused breathing.

1. Explain how stress can be described as a person's mental and emotional reactions to a situation.

2. What is the quickest way to neutralize the stress response?

Turning Stress into Strength
Lecture 14—Transcript

Welcome back. We have already learned about the stress hormones adrenaline, aldosterone, and cortisol. We have reviewed the research on how acute and chronic stress can make us sick. Today, we will start to look at biologic interventions that will actually help us turn stress into strength.

Remember, stress is almost always an emotional reaction to a situation. It is how we respond. Stress impacts our ability to think clearly, to respond appropriately, and even to perform at our best. Our stress level impacts not only how we feel at the end of the day, it impacts our health, and even our relationships, because quite frankly, no one really enjoys being around a stressed-out person.

I majored in English Literature, so I love literature, and I love quotes. Adyashanti is a teacher in Northern California, and he had this to say, "Suffering happens between the ears. Everything else is just a situation." And of course, one of the most famous authors, Mark Twain said, "I have suffered a great many misfortunes, most of which never happened." Both the quote by Adyashanti and Mark Twain tell us that what matters is how we see the world. In other words, through what lens do we see?

Now, we use these expressions all the time: "Oh, she sees through rose-colored glasses," or "Oh, he is a Debbie Downer." We say these kinds of things, but what does it mean to really see the world through rose-colored glasses? Or the more famous expression, is your glass half full, or is your glass half empty?

The way I teach it to my patients is like this: I tell my patients that frequently, you can't control the world around you. As a matter of fact, if you walk into my office, the first thing you see is the serenity prayer. And for those of you who are not familiar with it, basically what it says is, "God, give me the strength to know what things I can change and what things I can't, and the wisdom to know the difference." Frequently there are things we can't change; we can't control everything. We can't control our kids' every move, our spouse's every move, our boss, although we would like to, chances are we can't. So it is the initiating events that happen that we can't control. But what can we control? We can control our perception. Through what lens do we see those events? Let me give you a little vignette, a little example. Imagine a dad rushing off to work, and has to drop his kid off to school. They get in the car, dad is driving, and all of the sudden the train has to go by, so the arm goes down, and the car can't move. Dad is sitting there all tense behind the wheel, and little Johnny next to him says, "Wow, dad, we get to see a train." Two people see the same exact thing with totally different perception. That is the difference between reducing the stress hormones, which dad was doing, hanging onto the wheel, upset that he is late for work, and little Johnny, who is really thrilled to see the train.

So it is our perception that leads to the physical response and the effect that we talked about when we release the stress hormones.

So remember, stress is not the situation, but your mental and emotional reaction to it. Let's take a look at a research study that beautifully illustrates the connection between how we see the world through what lens we see, and health.

This is one of my absolute favorite studies. I have a lot of favorite studies, but this is a good one. This is the Mother Theresa study. Students were asked to watch a movie about Mother Theresa's activity, so they got to see Mother Theresa administering to the sick, taking care of the poor, the downtrodden, and so on. A protein that protects the body from infection, called IgA, was measured. Now, in a majority of the students, 92 percent, this protein went up, this protective protein increased. But, in about eight percent of the students, their immune system was affected in the negative. Their IgA level went down after watching the movie about Mother Theresa. The researchers did not stop there, the students were then asked to write a story about a photo of a couple on a park bench, and all they got to see was the backs of the couple, man and a woman, sitting on a park bench. They were asked to make up a story. I do this with my patients all the time. So the students came up with stories like this: He is proposing; they are getting married; they are going to have a baby. That was some of the students. But that other eight percent whose immune system went down when they watched the Mother Theresa movie had these kinds of stories: She distrusts him; he is manipulating her; they are abandoning each other. These were the same students who had a reduction in their IgA while watching Mother Theresa. In other words, these students saw everything in the negative. Their glass was half empty. They were not seeing through rose-colored glasses. In fact, when they were questioned, they really disliked Mother Theresa. They wanted nothing to do with taking care of the sick and poor in India. Actually, it annoyed them, and their immune system showed us that. But what is even more interesting about this study, the researchers went back and looked at who were the sickest students over the previous year, and you got it, that is right, it was those students that had the negative response to the Mother Theresa movie, and those students who wrote the stories about abandonment and manipulation that were sick all the time.

These researchers concluded that perception was the key. How you see the world. Now, one of the things I tell my patients is this: Can you change your environment, get rid of your spouse, get rid of your kids, get rid of your boss, get rid of your job, go and put yourself on a deserted island? Chances are none of us can do that. But what can we do? We can change how we react to, and perceive, our environment.

Charles Darwin had this to say. Darwin said, "It's not the strongest of the species that survives, nor the most intelligent, but it is actually the one that is most responsive to change." So how do we change? For those of you who are thinking, "I see everything negative," do not give up. We all can change. So we need to learn a couple of simple techniques. How do we learn how to respond to stress differently, in a way that actually negates the effect of the stress hormones? In a moment, I will give you a simple technique that will help you do just that.

But first, I need you to do a little exercise, and you might want to get a paper and pen for this if you can, if you can't, you can do the exercise later. But, I would like if you would take a piece of paper and divide the paper into fours, four quadrants. On the left-hand side of the sheet, I want you to write stress zone. On the right-hand side, I want you to write stress-free zone. Now, take a look at your x-axis. The x-axis on the left, I want you to label negative emotions. And on the right, I want you to label that side positive emotions. Now let's take the y-axis, up on the north position I want you to write adrenaline, sympathetic nervous system, stimulating nervous system ready to go. That is your adrenaline emotion. On the bottom of the y-axis I want you to write relaxation, low-energy low arousal. So you got it? Negative is on the left, positive is on the right.

So now I want you to start to think about the kinds of emotions you feel throughout the day. Every one of us lives in these four quadrants. I want you to begin to think about when you were on the left, and when you were on the right, and we are going to take a look at how this works. Now, I know I want to live on the right all the time, because that is where all the positive emotions are sitting, but there is a good chance that I do not spend all my time there, but I can work on it. And that is what this is about.

So let's take the paper and go up to the upper left quadrant. Remember now, these are negative emotions, because we are on the left, and they are high-energy so think about what are some high energy negative emotions? And they may be emotions that you have felt, may be even in the last 24 hours, or emotions you felt sometime in your life. And if you have not felt any, well that is good, but put a few down anyway.

So, high-energy negative emotions. The first one I can think of is hate. That is a high-energy negative emotion. The second one I think about is fear, and I will tell you fear is the opposite of love. Envy, anger, and frustration, these are just a few examples of high-energy negative emotions. And remember, I talked about anger in the previous lecture, and said anger increases the risk of a heart attack 230 percent. There is another personality type that I have to mention in here that keeps company with anger, and that is hostility. And the hostile personality type also increases the risk of cardiac events. So we have our upper left quadrant.

Let's go to the lower left quadrant, now we are in our low energy zone, this is our relaxation zone, but because we are on the left, we are looking for low-energy negative emotions. What might some of these be? I will bet some of you are writing down or thinking about things like, "I feel depressed," or "I feel lonely." Maybe even sad, or hopeless. These are our low-energy negative emotions.

So the left side of our page has negative emotions high and low. Now let's keep going counter-clockwise, let's cross over to the right side, and let's take a look at some low-energy positive emotions. What might these be? I always write on my list compassion. I also like to write empathy. I think we can even consider contentment, for example, a low-energy positive emotion. I feel content. And even sympathy.

Now we head up to the power zone, the upper right quadrant. These are our high-energy positive emotions, and I bet you can come up with a lot of them. For me, the four I come up with are joy, victory, courage, feeling courageous, and of course love.

So all day long, we are moving between these four quadrants, and our goal is to make a list of the emotions that we experience, to write them down, and then look at how much time am I spending on the left side of this page? And even more importantly, how can I get myself over to the right? Now I do not expect you to go from feeling hate for someone to feeling love for someone in 10 seconds. If you can do that, that is great, but what I want to do is when you are feeling that hate, or that anger, I want to at least get you to neutral, which is back to that y-axis, I want to get you back to neutral and I am going to show you how to do that. Because if you find yourself experiencing negative thoughts, having negative emotions, it is literally important to know how do I flip the switch? How do I turn the key on this and shift the thought and thereby shift the consequence of the stress hormones?

Now there is something else I have to add to this story. We talked a lot about the negative, we talked about the glass being half empty instead of half full, we are talking about the negative impact of stress, let's go to the positive. What about positive emotions? What about people who have positive thoughts all the time, the optimists of the world? The people who see the world through a half full glass? What does the research show?

Well this is what it shows. Those people have increased longevity. Positive emotions reduce morbidity from various diseases. This greatly affects our mind. Positive emotions result in us having what is called more cognitive flexibility. We are more creative. We are better at problem solving. We are more innovative. All of these things are increased when we experience positive emotions, and as you will see in a minute, I do not want you to just think a positive emotion, I do not want you to think victory, I do not want you to think love, I want you to feel them, I want you to feel love. That is what has the effect on your body. Positive emotions even improve our job performance. They make us do everything better. We think better, we think clearer, we are happier; we see the world through a different set of lenses.

Now, I have some patients who see the world through the negative. And sometimes the first thing I have to do is tell them, "I want you to keep a gratefulness journal," and we will talk more about that in later lectures. But their job is at night to write down things that they are grateful for, because I want them to start feeling love and getting the physiologic benefit of the positive emotion.

When you are in a stressful situation, or you are thinking negative thoughts, the first thing I want you to do is neutralize the negative thoughts and feelings. I call this taking a time out. We do this with children all the time. Children are running around screaming, hitting, fighting, what do we say? "Take a time out." The kid knows what this means, they have to go and sit down; they have to take a few deep breaths and take it easy. Children know what taking a time out means. I want you to take a time out before you say something you are going to regret, or before you do something you are going to regret. So how do we do this?

One of my favorite breathing techniques to neutralize stress, I learned from my colleagues at Heart Math. Of course I love it because I am a cardiologist, and it is all about the heart. It is called the Heart Focused Breath, or Heart Focused Breathing. How does it work? Breathing controls our autonomic nervous system. When we take a big breath in, our heart rate goes up; when we exhale, our heart rate goes down. But if we breathe in a cyclic rhythmical way it stabilizes our autonomic nervous system. It takes our foot off the gas.

Now let's practice this for a minute, and this will be a little bit of an experience for some people. If you are driving the car, this may not be a good time to practice this because it will relax you, so you may want to come back to this later on. The first thing you do is you take that time out. Sometimes we have to remove ourselves from the stressful situation. Sometimes we, literally, physically have to leave the room. I am about to say something I am going to regret, I am going to do something really stupid, I am going to kick the wall, whatever it is, we have to neutralize that emotion. So the first thing I want you to do is to take a breath. Most of us breathe from the upper third of our lungs. I want you to take a breath that in yoga is called a yogic breath. I want you to take a breath for five seconds in, and five seconds out. I just want you to experience that, before we go to the first step. Five seconds in, and five seconds out. I bet your body is already starting to relax. So now you have taken your time out, you stopped yourself from saying what you are going to regret.

Now I am going to ask you to take the longest journey you will ever have to take, and it is 18 inches. I want you to get out of your head and I want you to drop your focus down to your heart. I want you to imagine that you are breathing in and out through your heart. This may feel funny at first, but in a few minutes you are going to see that it becomes really easy. We call this heart breathing. Five seconds in, five seconds out. Five seconds in, and five seconds out. And if you are somewhere where you can do this, I invite you to try it right now, because when I have my patients do this, the first thing they say is, "Oh, I feel more relaxed." Sometimes when people show up in my office and they come rushing in, and the first thing we do is we put them on the scale and weigh them. Well, guess what that does to their blood pressure? They look at their weight, they know Dr. G. is coming in and they are thinking, "Oh my God, I am in trouble," their blood pressure goes up. So I come into the room and here's a high blood pressure reading. So is my first reaction to give a blood pressure pill? No. The first thing I do is of course re-check the blood pressure, but before I do that, I have my patient start to breathe five seconds in, and five seconds out.

The minute you start the breath, it interrupts the body's stress response. It just tells that train to halt, stop, and literally it stops, right in its tracks. If you are having trouble doing this for the first time, you may want to use a little trick that we teach, which is to actually place your hand over your heart. Place your right hand over your heart, and if it is comfortable, place your left hand over your right hand, and begin to breathe in and out. You may also find that closing your eyes at first will make this easier, so try it again. Five seconds in, and five seconds out.

With practice, you will be able to do this with your eyes open or your eyes closed, either way. But guess what? If you are walking into a board meeting, or you are feeling stressed out about meeting with your boss, you now know how, even with your eyes wide open, to control your autonomic nervous system simply by using your breath.

Now there is another important piece to this exercise. So let's say you have a problem, we have all had this. We have a problem that we are trying to solve and we can't get the solution, and we are going around and around and around, we can't get the solution.

So I want you to do this, I want you first, before we do the next section, to think about something that elicits a positive emotion in you. Remember we wrote some of those down; so think about something that makes you feel love, or appreciation. I bet I can guess what a few are. Maybe it is your little puppy. Maybe your puppy elicits that love feeling. I definitely know it is your new grandbaby, and it certainly is your baby. Stay away from people like your spouse, because even though we love them, sometimes it is mixed. I want you to get that unconditional love feeling, or appreciation, a big feeling of gratefulness that comes from the heart.

So now while you are doing your breathing, five seconds in and five seconds out, through your heart, I want you to add the power of the positive emotion. We already saw that the positive emotions are good for us, they improve our cognition, they increase our mental flexibility, and they help us to make decisions. One of the easiest ways to do this step is to remember a special place, someone you love or appreciate, and I said to myself when I first did this, "I am going to put my nephew there, my niece there, and my little poodle there." All of these, for me, elicit the love emotion. Now remember, I do not want you to just think the emotion, I do not want you to think love, I want you to feel love.

So let's review the steps. Step one, is the heart-focused breath, we bring our focus down to our heart, we have already taken our time out, right? Removing myself from the situation, dropping my focus down to my heart. And then number two; I am going to start my breathing, five seconds in, five seconds out. And then I am going to add in the power of the positive emotion, I am going to think about my baby, my grandbaby, my puppy, whatever it is that elicits a love or appreciation reaction. And then what I want you to do is I want you to hold that feeling of appreciation or love for about 20 seconds. I want you to hold that exact feeling, see that grandbaby in your arms, then I want you to radiate that love to yourself, and to all those around you. And I can tell you at the end of the day, this is how we are going to change the world.

Remember, do not just think positive, be positive, feel positive. And when you catch your mind wandering away, can't keep the focus, do not be upset, just focus back on the breathing, always bring yourself back to the breath, so when the grocery list gets in the way, focus on the breathing. Five seconds in, five seconds out, reconnect with the feelings of caring, love, and appreciation. And if you have a problem that you have not been able to solve, or solve with your mind, now I want you to ask your heart, "Give me a better solution to this situation." And I guarantee it; your heart is going to speak.

I promise you if you practice this technique, you are going to stop saying things that you regret. You are no longer going to be the angry person, the person that people like to stand clear of. Not only that, you are going to neutralize the negative impact of stress on your body, and you will get all the benefits of the positive emotions.

Today, we reviewed our emotional landscape, we discussed the power of positive emotions, and we learned a powerful technique to neutralize stress. And remember the power of your own breath, because your breath has the power to heal.

Meditation, Yoga, and Guided Imagery
Lecture 15

Ma ore hospitals and medical clinics than ever before are educating their patients about the benefits of meditation, yoga, and guided imagery and are using these tools to lower blood pressure, decrease anxiety, decrease blood sugar, and even improve surgical outcomes in their patients. In this lecture, you will explore some of the research on these mind-body techniques and look at how they are shifting the paradigm of Western medicine and revolutionizing the way doctors and hospitals care for their patients.

The Benefits of Meditation
- The negative effects of stress on our bodies are endless. If we do not do something to change our response to stress, the end result is high blood pressure, diabetes, high cholesterol, and even heart attack and stroke. Relaxation practices such as meditation and yoga can help you react better to stress.

- Meditation is the skillful, sustained, applied use of attention. The attention can be on your breath—breathing in and breathing out—or it can be on a word, but regardless of what you choose to focus on, your attention is focused.

- You may think that sitting quietly would be easy, but try to do it for five minutes and focus on only one thing. You will find that your mind jumps around from thought to thought. It takes practice to control your mind.

- A meditation practice may be formal or informal. The two most common forms of formal meditation that are used in health care are mindfulness-based stress reduction, which comes out of the Buddhist tradition, and transcendental meditation, which comes out of the Vedic tradition.

- Meditation can also be performed as an informal practice. You can informally practice meditation at any time any day. Whenever you get a free moment, take five longer, deeper breaths—five seconds in and five seconds out.

- You want to have a balanced autonomic nervous system, and techniques such as transcendental meditation, mindfulness, yoga, and others impact the autonomic nervous system, stopping the stress process.

Research on Meditation
- In 1995, a study that was published in the *Journal of Hypertension* was conducted of 127 African Americans with very high, difficult-to-control blood pressure. The patients that were randomized to the meditation group were taught transcendental meditation. They were given a mantra, and they practiced meditation for 20 minutes twice a day. These individuals were able to drop their systolic blood pressure by 10.7 millimeters of mercury.

- Research also shows that people who learn to meditate have a statistically significant reduction in anxiety. They feel less stressed, less anxious, and less worried. Transcendental meditation has even been shown to decrease insulin resistance.

- When people begin to meditate, there is a reduction in addictive behaviors, such as cigarette smoking and alcohol use. We are just starting to understand the biochemistry of the brain, which might explain these effects, through functional MRI imaging.

The Benefits of Yoga
- The word "yoga" means "yoke" or "union," which refers to the true integration, or union, of body, mind, and spirit. Yoga has been around for thousands of years; it is an ancient form of optimal living that is a very large part of Ayurvedic medicine.

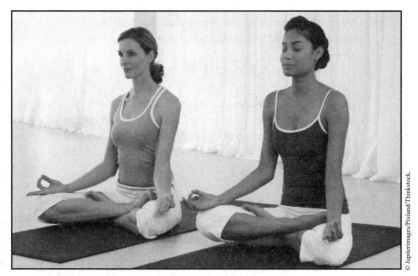

Research shows that relaxation practices—such as meditation and yoga—are effective at managing the stress response.

- Yoga is a lifestyle approach that ties together physical, mental, emotional, and spiritual aspects of healing. The most common aspects of yoga are stretching and meditation. The yoga postures are called asanas.

- There are many misconceptions about yoga: It is not only for the flexible or fit, it is not a religion, and you do not have to be in good health to do it. You might want to modify some of the poses and stretches because you don't want to do any that might hurt you, but there are many poses and stretches that everyone can do—including just sitting in a chair.

- Yoga enhances relaxation and increases parasympathetic tone. In other words, it puts you in a state of relaxation. It decreases the sympathetic nervous system, lowers blood pressure, and improves serum lipids, cholesterol, and triglycerides.

- Yoga can benefit any ailment that you might have, including anxiety, arthritis, asthma, fibromyalgia, headaches, and high blood pressure.

- You are not expected to learn yoga right away. With your physician's permission, you might want to buy a gentle yoga tape and start to try some simple exercises—or you might go to a yoga class. There are integrative medicine centers all over the world that offer yoga and meditation. However, you can probably do the breathing exercises right away.

Research on Mantra Repetition

- Mantras have been extensively studied. They offer an easy way to stop your mind from jumping around from one thought to another. In addition, your mind worries about things that happened in the past and everything that will happen in the future.

- A mantra is a sacred word, chant, or sound that is repeated over and over again. The goal of a mantra is to cultivate inner peace. It could be the repetition of a word such as "shalom," "Rama," or any other word from another spiritual tradition. In its most literal sense, the word "mantra" means "to free from the mind."

- Heart rate variability is the beat-to-beat change in our heart's rate, and it is an indicator of nervous system function. Research shows that low heart rate variability is predictive of having a heart attack and sudden death.

- The breathing technique that you have been introduced to can improve heart rate variability. Research conducted at the Scripps Center for Integrative Medicine showed that heart rate variability can be improved in people with congestive heart failure by using breathing techniques and associated mantras.

- Jill Bormann studied the power of mantra in people who have post-traumatic stress disorder (PTSD). Her research showed statistically significant reductions in all the major variables related to post-traumatic stress disorder when participants consistently practiced a mantra.

- When you are feeling angry, anxious, upset, or afraid, repeating a mantra can help calm you down. It is also a great technique if you have trouble falling asleep.

Guided Imagery

- Guided imagery is a program of directed thoughts that guide your imagination to a relaxed, focused state. It is based on the concept that your body and mind are connected. Using all of your senses, your body seems to respond as though what you are imagining is real.

- Studies have shown that guided imagery can statistically reduce stress and anxiety. Some physicians use guided imagery with patients before and after surgery because research shows a reduction in pain medicine, surgical complications, and recovery time in the hospital.

Questions to Consider

1. Name three health benefits of yoga and meditation.

2. Where has guided imagery proven to be of value in health care?

Meditation, Yoga, and Guided Imagery
Lecture 15—Transcript

More and more hospitals and medical clinics are educating their patients about the benefits of meditation, yoga, and guided imagery. I remember years ago when we started a yoga and meditation program at Scripps Center for Integrative Medicine. This was in the 1990s and the administration use to call it Dr. Guarneri's cult. At the Scripps Center for Integrative Medicine, we have been using yoga, meditation and guided imagery for just about everything; to lower blood pressure, to decrease anxiety, to decrease blood sugar, and even to improve surgical outcomes.

Today we will explore some of the research on these mind-body techniques and look at how they are actually shifting the paradigm of western medicine. So why would a cardiologist be interested in things like meditation and yoga? For one, research is proving these practices are incredibly effective at managing the stress response.

Let's review what happens when we are under stress. We talked about the stress hormones, adrenaline, aldosterone, and cortisol and for a cardiologist this is a big deal because everything I treat every day is impacted by the stress hormones. If the stress hormones are high or if our foot is on the gas all the time, this increases our blood lipids, especially our triglycerides. Remember I talked about it making our blood sticky. If we have sticky blood or activated platelets as it is called, we are more prone to have a heart attack. Stress hormones increase, blood pressure, increase blood sugar, and the list is endless. But, for my heart patients, I see something else that is very common: When people are under stress they have more chest discomfort, what is called angina, because the stress hormones cause the arteries to constrict. They squeeze shut.

Now I did not even mention all of the other aspects of stress—things like cognitive function, osteoporosis, we talked about all of those. If we do not do something to change our response to stress the end result is what I see every day in my practice, high blood pressure, diabetes, high cholesterol, and even heart attack and stroke. This is why, as a cardiologist, I had to expand my toolbox to include many of these practices. Let's begin with meditation and yoga, which we have been teaching at Scripps to our patients and guess what also our staff since 1996.

There are many definitions of meditation, but I am going to give you one that is short and to the point. Meditation is the skillful, sustained, applied use of attention. The attention can be on the breath, breathing in and breathing out. It can be on a word, but it is attention focused. You may think that sounds easy. I invite you to sit for just five minutes, not right now, but when you have a quiet moment, and just focus on your breathing for five minutes. I am breathing in and breathing out and you will see what happens to your mind. Your mind jumps, jumps, jumps, jumps from thought to thought. It takes practice to control the mind.

A meditation practice may be formal or informal. The two most common forms of meditation used in health-care, those with the greatest amount of research are mindfulness-based stress reduction which comes out of the Buddhist tradition and transcendental meditation which comes out of the Vedic tradition. Transcendental meditation, for example, teaches a formal practice. Students are encouraged to sit 20 minutes two times a day and focus on a word or a mantra every day.

Now there is something called an informal practice. I invite you to start the informal practice today. We do this with our patients all the time. What do we do all day? We look at our watch. How many times a day do you look at your watch? Take a green dot and put it right on the face of your watch, and now when you look at your watch you are going to take what you call a mini moment. When you see that green dot this is your clue to take five longer, deeper breaths. We have learned about the five second breath. Five seconds in, five seconds out. Just take longer, deeper breaths; even just do five. Immediately you will negate your stress hormones, as we have already discussed, and you will feel your body going into a more relaxed position.

Now we talked about the autonomic nervous system, and it is worth mentioning again here. It's that seesaw effect. Remember autonomic means automatic. We have a sympathetic component that is stimulating and ready to go and we have a parasympathetic component that is relaxing. Again our foot is either on the gas or our foot is on the brake and really what we want to do is we want to have a balanced autonomic nervous system. You can't have your foot on the brake all day because you never get up and do anything. We already saw that if you had your foot on the gas all day, you are going to get really sick. Well techniques like TM meditation, transcendental meditation, mindfulness, yoga, and others impact the autonomic nervous system just like the breath, just taking the five second in, five second out breath, stops the stress process.

A fascinating study was done in 1995. This was a study that was conducted in African-Americans with very high, difficult to control blood pressure. It was published in the Journal of Hypertension. There were 127 patients in this study and I want to focus on those that got randomized to the meditation group. They were taught transcendental meditation. They were given a mantra, and they practiced with their mantra and their meditation 20 minutes two times a day. What they found was these individuals with hard to control high blood pressure were able to drop the systolic blood pressure by 10.7 millimeters of mercury. That could be the difference between needing a blood pressure medicine and not needing blood pressure medicine at all.

What else does the research show? People who learn to meditate have a statistically significant reduction in anxiety. They feel less stressed, they feel less anxious, and they worry less. We talked a lot about natural treatments for diabetes. Well we have to add meditation to the list because transcendental meditation has been shown to decrease insulin resistance.

Something else very interesting happens when people begin to meditate. There is a reduction in cigarette smoking and there is even a reduction in alcohol use. You may wonder why, with meditation, you see a reduction in what we call addictive behaviors like smoking, alcohol, tobacco of all types, even cigars. There may be some really neat biochemistry going on in the brain with meditation. We are just starting to understand this through functional MRI imaging, but that is not today's subject and some day we will understand the nuances of all the brain changes that occur. I think it is deeper.

For me when I see my patients and they are eating too much food or they are drinking too much alcohol or they are using too much tobacco, I begin to wonder what is driving that train, and invariably they tell me it is stress. "I have 20 friends in this pack of cigarettes Dr. Guarneri." "That donut made me feel really good." And a very common one I hear is, "I had a stressful day. I went home and drank a bottle of wine just to unwind." I believe that what the meditation is doing here is, as people begin to meditate, they begin to find inner peace. They begin to feel more relaxed, more comfortable in their own body. If we are at peace we are less likely to say, "I need that cigarette to make me feel good," or, "I am going to eat that donut right now." That is why I think we see the reduction in a lot of the addictive behaviors.

At the Scripps Center for Integrative Medicine we teach yoga and meditation together so our patients learn both. Let's take a look at yoga. What does yoga mean? Yoga means "yoke" or "union." But what is being yoked? In yoga what we are referring to is the true integration or union, if you might, of body, mind, and spirit. Yoga has been around for thousands of years. It is an ancient form of optimal living and it is a very big part of Ayurvedic medicine.

Remember we talked about Ayurvedic medicine as being a global healing tradition. In holistic integrative medicine, physicians frequently use tools from Ayurvedic medicine for their patients. In this case it is yoga. Yoga is a lifestyle approach that ties together physical, mental, emotional, and spiritual aspects of healing. It includes many techniques, and there is even something called the eight-fold path which includes ethical living. But, for our purposes, the most common aspects of yoga are stretching and meditation.

We call the yoga postures asanas, but you can look at any football field, any Olympic stadium, and I guarantee you, you are going to see a lot of yoga poses because those poses are stretching. There are a lot of misconceptions about yoga. The first one I hear is, "Yoga is only for the flexible. I can't do that. You have to be flexible, you have to be fit." The other I hear is, "Yoga is a religious practice." The third is, "Yoga is only for those in good health." Well I want to clear away these misconceptions because yoga is not only for the flexible or fit, yoga is not a religion, and you do not have to be in good health.

I have been using yoga safely in my, sometimes very sick, heart patients for over 15 years and, yes, I might modify some of the poses and I do not want people to do stretches that might hurt them, but there are many, many poses and many stretches that everyone can do, including even sitting in a chair.

Let's look at some of the health benefits of yoga. For one, it enhances relaxation. It increases parasympathetic tone. In other words, it puts us in a state of relaxation. When I ask my patients, "Did you like the yoga class today?" they always say, "I feel so relaxed." It decreases that sympathetic nervous system. It helps us get our foot off the gas. On the cardiac side, it lowers blood pressure and improves serum lipids, cholesterol, and triglycerides. There are many health benefits, and there is a textbook by Dr. McCall called *Yoga as Medicine.* If you go through this book you will find that yoga can benefit any ailment that you might have whether it is anxiety, arthritis, asthma, fibromyalgia, headaches, and many of the ones we already mentioned like high blood pressure. Yoga will help.

I will tell you where it helps me the most. In the first lecture I mentioned that I put in a lot of stents, over 700 stents a year. When you are putting in a stent you stand over a patient wearing a leaded apron. I have to wear the lead to protect me because I am using radiation to look at someone's heart. After years of doing this, that heavy lead apron took a toll on my lumbar spine, on my lower back. This is very common. Many physicians stop practicing interventional cardiology for this exact reason.

I remember when I was advised by a surgeon to have three disks taken out of my back because I could not walk, from where I am standing now, 20 feet. I went to our yoga instructor Karen and I said, "Karen I need you to give me some postures that are going to relax the muscles in my back so that I can start to heal those disks that are shifting," and she did and I have never looked back. That was ten years ago. When my back acts up now, and it will sometimes, I always turn to yoga.

I also had another interesting experience in the 1990s. I mentioned that we conducted research with Dr. Dean Ornish and we took really sick heart patients and we taught them yoga and meditation. We got them exercising and for some people that was just simply walking barely around the track, but they got better as time went on. We put them on a low fat diet and I know the low fat diet is not for everyone, but in this study it was very low fat diet and we put people in support groups. We demonstrated that chest pain was reduced 91 percent. Now that is great medicine.

I have a lot of colleagues especially in the '90s that were very old school. Their thinking was what we call the reductionist approach. They wanted to know, what was the one thing that worked? Was it your exercise? Was it your yoga and meditation? Was it the diet? What is it that worked in these patients? I thought to myself when I was being questioned, this is really crazy. This is not a pill for cancer. We are talking about eating right, exercising, sitting in support groups, and doing yoga and meditation so how would it sound if I decided I am going to do the reductionist approach and I am going to tell one group of patients, "You can eat whatever you want, do not worry about your heart disease because you are going to walk," and tell the other group, "You do not have to do yoga and meditation, you are just going to exercise." It just did not make any sense.

There was a creative chap out there, Dr. Blumenthal, who decided to try to tease this out a little bit. He took 107 people with coronary disease and they wore heart monitors and what he was looking for was what is called ischemia, decreased blood flow to the heart muscle during mental stress. Then he trained them for four months in stress management, put part of the group in exercise, and this is my favorite part, the third group went to the usual care. That means they got to see their physician according to scheduled appointments. He followed these patients for five years and guess what he found? Those people who were in the usual care group did the worst. The people in the exercise group were in the middle in terms of cardiac events. The people in the stress management group had a 74 percent lower risk of cardiac events and decreased ischemia. He separated out some of the components and in this case the stress management group did the best. I do not expect you to learn yoga over night. With your physician's permission you may buy a gentle yoga tape and start to try some simple exercises or you might go to a yoga class. There are integrative medicine centers all over the country now that are offering yoga and meditation. I expect that you can do the breathing exercises right away. I am going to give you another little exercise that works as quickly.

This is a technique called mantra repetition. Mantras have been extensively studied. They offer an easy way to stop what is called "monkey mind." If you have never heard the expression of monkey mind, monkey mind is when we go from thought to thought to thought to thought, the way a monkey jumps from branch to branch to branch to branch; grocery list, shopping list, husband, spouse, partner, kids, pick up the kids from school, you know how the mind goes, oh, plus, I will worry about things that happened in the past and I will really worry about everything that will happen in the future. We can't turn it off.

A mantra is a sacred word, a chant, or a sound that is repeated over and over again. The goal of the mantra is to cultivate inner peace. It could be the repetition of a work like shalom, or Rama, and there are many others from every spiritual tradition. If you have a spiritual tradition you might want to find a word that can become your mantra. The word "mantra" in its most literal sense means "to free from the mind."

Before we look at the powerful research on mantra repetition, we need to first understand something called heart rate variability. Now this is a tough concept for a lot of people to get. Heart rate variability is the beat to beat change in our heart's rate. It is not our heart rate; it is the beat to beat change and the timing literally between the beats. It represents the body's ability to speed up and slow down efficiently. This is what keeps us flexible and, quite frankly, healthy. If your heart was not able to speed up, you would not be able to run up a flight of steps and if it did not slow down, you certainly would not be able to sleep.

Why is it so important in cardiology? Heart rate variability is an indicator of our nervous system function. If your heart rate variability is low, that means your autonomic nervous system is less flexible. That places you at high cardiac risk. If your heart rate variability is high, you are at lower cardiac risk. The research shows that low heart rate variability is predictive of having a heart attack and sudden death.

I taught you a breathing technique, remember? The five seconds in, five seconds out. Well that breathing technique can improve heart rate variability, just learning how to breathe. We conducted research at Scripps where we showed that we can improve heart rate variability in people with congestive heart failure. That is important. It can be modified. One of my favorite studies to demonstrate how heart rate variability can be modified was published in the *British Medical Journal* in 2001. In this study, people were asked to either do repetitive prayer, in this case it was the Rosary, or pick a sacred word and do mantra repetition. Both practices demonstrated a decrease in sympathetic tone and an increase in heart rate variability.

Could this be why, in every spiritual tradition you can think of, there is some form of repetitive prayer. I was raised Catholic so we had the rosary. Buddhists have what is called a mala, 108 beads. Hindus do repetitive prayer. Every spiritual tradition, for some reason, has chosen repetitive prayer. What I have found in my practice that when you are doing repetitive prayer or you are saying your mantra your mind is not on the past and it is not worrying about the future. It keeps us in the present moment. I do ask my patients to pick a mantra, and I give them a list. I give them a list that comes out of the work of a researcher named Jill Bormann.

Jill Bormann studied the power of mantra in people who have post traumatic stress disorder, people who were coming back from war, Vietnam War in this case, and could not turn off the memories of the battles. They could not sleep. They would sit up all night, all sorts of medical problems. She just had them pick a mantra and to practice it all the time. But she told these Vets, she said, "I want you to use that mantra all the time except for when you have to do something like calculate a mathematics problem, otherwise the only thing I want you to do is the mantra. If your mind goes back to Vietnam do the mantra, your mind goes back to the past do the mantra." What did she find?

Her research showed statistically significant reductions in all the major variables related to post traumatic stress disorder. When I give my patients the mantra list, I tell them when you are walking, jogging, do your mantra because I would rather have them doing their mantra instead of saying, "I am going to get revenge on so and so," and, "Something bad happened ten years ago and I just can't get it out of my mind." When we are thinking those thoughts, guess what? It could have happened ten years ago, but if you are feeling that anger you are just producing stress hormones, so I ask my patients to do the mantra when they are walking, jogging, waiting in lines.

I will tell you when I do my mantra. When I get into one of those voice loops that takes you forever to get out of; that is when I get really impatient so I just let the voice loop go and I do my mantra. When you are feeling angry it will calm you down, anxious, upset, or afraid. One of the best techniques before a young doctor goes to give their first presentation is I have them breathe and then if they happen to have a mantra I have them begin to repeat it. It is a great technique if you have trouble falling asleep. When you are trying to get to sleep and feeling like I just can't get there start to say your mantra over and over again. Your mind is going to start wandering, you are going to start worrying, take it back to the mantra over and over. I guarantee it: You will fall asleep.

We have now seen a few of the powerful tools which are available and at our fingertips to neutralize stress. Meditation and yoga are powerful medicine. Mantra repetition and prayer are powerful medicine. Now let's take a look at one additional tool that I use every day in my practice and that tool is guided imagery. Guided imagery is a program of directed thoughts that guide your imagination to a relaxed, focused state. It is based on the concept that your body and mind are connected. Using all of your senses, your body seems to respond as though what you are imagining is real.

Studies have shown that guided imagery can significantly reduce stress and anxiety. We use it all the time. We use guided imagery at Scripps before patients go to surgery and after surgery. Why? Because the research shows a reduction in pain, less pain medicine, less surgical complications and a two day shorter stay in the hospital. That's amazing medicine.

As we come to the end of our time together, remember there are many paths to stress reduction. Find a path that works for you. We have explored a few: the power of meditation, yoga, mantra repetition, prayer, and guided imagery. Research shows that meditation, yoga, and guided imagery are powerful tools. These are tools that you can implement immediately. But even beyond this, the powerful synergy between these tools and Western medicine is revolutionizing the way doctors and hospitals are caring for their patients.

Natural Approaches to Mental Health
Lecture 16

In this lecture, you will explore some of the research on antidepressant medication and learn about what people can do to improve their mental health naturally. Research clearly demonstrates that a diet of low-glycemic foods, whole grains, and omega-3 fatty acids is associated with a lower rate of depression and bipolar disorder. Depression can also be improved by replacing missing nutrients, such as vitamin D and magnesium, and by adding supplements, such as SAM-e and Saint-John's-wort. In addition, people with depression should get out into the sunlight and exercise.

Macronutrition and Well-Being

- The human brain needs a balance of nutrients to maintain a positive mood, and if it does not get all of the nutrients it requires, it does not work correctly.

- The human brain is fueled by molecules, which come from our diet, and just as in the case with the rest of our body, some of the foods we eat promote brain health while others may actually cause harm.

- Modern psychiatry uses some molecules to alter brain function— mainly in the form of medication, such as antidepressants. However, in general, modern psychiatry tends to ignore the molecules that we eat every day.

- The micronutrients that are important in brain function include the B vitamins (folate and B12), calcium and chromium, minerals like magnesium and zinc, and antioxidants like vitamin E and selenium.

- Altering the micronutrients that are found in our food supply can have an effect on our brain's health. Processing food removes essential vitamins and nutrients from it, so make sure that you are eating whole foods. Folic acid, which is essential to brain health, is found in whole grains.

- Trans fats, processed vegetable oils, alcohol, and sugar impair a very important enzyme called delta-6 desaturase, which forms omega-3 fatty acids. The blocking of this enzyme by trans fats, processed vegetable oils, alcohol, and sugar causes the body to not be able to make essential omega-3s. Mounting evidence now links omega-3 deficiency in humans to a number of disorders, including depression and bipolar disorder.

- The Avon Longitudinal Study of Parents and Children demonstrated that a diet of lots of vegetables, fruit, fish, and grains was associated with a lower rate of depression and anxiety.

- A prospective study of over 10,000 adults was conducted to assess the links between the Mediterranean diet and depression. The Mediterranean diet is high in fruit, legumes, beans, lentils, green leafy vegetables, and fish, is low in saturated fat, and uses the good source of oil—olive oil. Of the people that were followed, the more fruits, nuts, legumes, and monounsaturated fats that were consumed, the less depression there was.

- There also appears to be a link between depression and bipolar disorder to diets with a high glycemic index, which are diets that are high in simple sugars and simple carbohydrates. Of the 691 women that were studied, 23 were diagnosed with bipolar disorder. In the *Journal of Affective Disorders*, researchers concluded that bipolar disorder was linked to diets with a high glycemic index.

- Food sensitivity causes a number of symptoms, including gas, bloating, arthritis, joint pain, skin rashes, and even mood changes. Food sensitivity has also been implicated in neurologic disorders of unknown cause.

- Gluten sensitivity is known to cause neurologic problems— particularly seizures in people who otherwise have no medical problems. According to a study published in *The Lancet* in 1996, gluten sensitivity is a contributing factor in schizophrenia, bipolar disorder, and anxiety.

Micronutrition and Well-Being

- When it comes to mental well-being, micronutrients, including vitamins and minerals, appear to be equally as important as macronutrients—the proteins and fats that are found in the foods that we eat.

- The problem of being deficient in magnesium, which comes mainly from green leafy vegetables, is widespread. A study that evaluated the link between diet and depression in over 5,000 people found an inverse correlation between magnesium intake in the diet and depression scores.

- Vitamin D, which is very important to bone health, affects so many different mechanisms and systems in our body. A 2005 study showed that low levels of 25-hydroxy vitamin D are significantly associated with a higher depression score. Another study found that psychiatric patients had significantly lower levels of vitamin D than a control group.

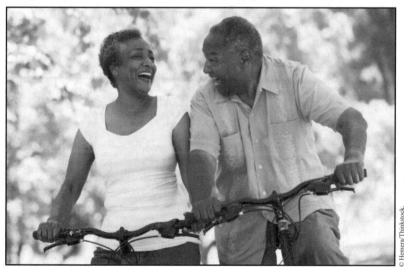

Riding bicycles outside is a great exercise activity that can help people who are depressed.

- Folate, a B vitamin, is one of the most important vitamins for treating depression. Folate can be used to treat depression with or without antidepressants. When folate is taken with an antidepressant medication such as Prozac, research shows that there is an improvement in depression beyond the effect of the antidepressant alone.

- Exercise is another treatment for depression. The problem is that many depressed people do not feel like exercising. An hour per day of exercise is recommended for people with or without depression, but a person who is depressed should at least start with 15 or 20 minutes of exercise per day and slowly increase the time.

- SAM-e is a potent antidepressant that should be taken under a physician's guidance because the dose has to be increased slowly over time—starting at about 200 milligrams per day and possibly increasing to 800 milligrams per day. One of the side effects of SAM-e is that it can produce a manic state, so people that have bipolar disorder—which is a combination of depression and mania—or a family history of bipolar disorder should not take SAM-e.

- Saint-John's-wort is almost as common an herbal remedy for mild to moderate depression as Prozac and Paxil are pharmaceutical remedies. The research shows that Saint-John's-wort might not be as effective for severe depression.

- For mild to moderate depression, 900 milligrams per day of Saint-John's-wort is a good option. However, depending on the preparation, Saint-John's-wort can interact with a long list of medications, so consult an integrative holistic physician before taking it.

- Nothing is better for depression than exercising in the sunlight. There are some people that live in areas where they do not get a lot of sun—particularly in the winter—and light therapy can help.

- In Canada, 100 patients with depression in the winter months—called seasonal affective disorder (SAD)—were treated with either Prozac or exposure to light. Depression improved equally in both groups, but those receiving light therapy had a faster response to that improvement. The authors concluded that light therapy is as good as the standard antidepressant approach with fewer side effects and much less overall risk.

Questions to Consider

1. Name two nonpharmaceutical approaches to depression.

2. Name two micronutrients that are linked to depression.

Natural Approaches to Mental Health
Lecture 16—Transcript

Americans spent 10 billion dollars on antidepressant and 14 billion dollars on antipsychotic medication in 2010. Medications like Paxil and Prozac have become household words. Today we will explore some of the research on antidepressant medication and look at what we can do to improve our mental health naturally.

We have seen a trend in modern psychiatry towards what we call polypharmacy. What does this mean? Polypharmacy means prescribing multiple medications for the so-called same diagnosis. Of over 13,000 psychiatric visits, which were monitored between 1996 and 2006, visits in which patients were given two or more psychiatric medications increased from 42 percent to 60 percent. We currently have 1.2 million children on two or more psychiatric medications. Is there any evidence to support the liberal use of these psychiatric medications in the majority of the population?

Let's take a look at some research. The STEP Bipolar Disorder study was a study to assess the relapse of bipolar disorder; 1469 patients with a diagnosis of bipolar disorder were given state of the art pharmaceutical therapy. They got the best that medicine can give and in spite of this state of the art pharmaceutical therapy the relapse rate at two years was 48.5 percent. A 2010 meta-analysis appeared in the *Journal of the American Medical Association* looking at antidepressants and depression. The authors concluded, and I quote, "The magnitude of benefit of antidepressant medication compared with placebo … may be minimal or nonexistent in patients with mild to moderate symptoms." Now for patients with the most severe depression these drugs seem to be of benefit, but for the majority of people with mild to moderate depression they may be no better than placebo.

The treatment of depression is complex. It can't simply be handled most of the time by a pill. I am not against antidepressant medication especially in people with severe depression, but what else can we do to enhance the treatment of depression beyond what clearly is the "ill to the pill" mentality.

To begin to address the question we must remember that the human brain is fueled by molecules. These molecules come from our diet and just as in the case with the rest of our body some of the foods we eat will promote brain health and others may actually cause harm.

If our brain does not get all of the nutrients it requires, quite simply, it doesn't work right. Modern psychiatry uses some molecules to alter brain function, mainly in the form of medication like the antidepressants Prozac and Celexa, just to name a few. But modern psychiatry tends to ignore the molecules that we eat every day. Remember what we said early on in the Science of Natural Healing, food is medicine and food is information.

The micronutrients that are important in brain function include things like the B vitamins, folate and B12, calcium and chromium, minerals like magnesium and zinc, and antioxidants like vitamin E and selenium and this is just naming a few. We have already discussed how processing food removes essential vitamins and nutrients from the food that we eat. For example, folic acid is essential to brain health. It is found in whole grains, but yet if we take a whole grain and we turn that whole grain into a bleached flour, we lose 67 percent of the folic acid. We also lose 85 percent of the magnesium and 50 to 60 percent of the B vitamins so altering our food supply, altering the micronutrients can have an effect on our brain's health.

What else can we eat that can infect our mood? Well, trans fats, processed vegetable oils, alcohol, and sugar impair a very important enzyme. This enzyme is called the delta-6 desaturase enzyme. It is an important enzyme in the body forming omega-3 fatty acids. Without this enzyme or the blocking of this enzyme from trans fats, processed vegetable oils, sugar—and remember alcohol is a sugar—the body can't make the essential omega-3s. Mounting evidence now links omega-3 deficiency in humans to a number of disorders, including depression and bipolar disorder.

Let's take a look at some of the mounting evidence. The Avon Longitudinal Study assessed the nutritional habits and mood of women at 32 weeks of pregnancy. The study concluded that a lower maternal intake of omega-3, in this case seafood, was linked to depression. A second study included 1046 women between the ages of 23 to 93. This study also looked at diet and depression. What it demonstrated was that a diet of lots of vegetables, fruit, fish, and grains was associated with a lower rate of depression and also anxiety.

A large prospective study of over 10,000 adults was conducted to assess for links between the Mediterranean diet and depression. We reviewed the Mediterranean diet, but let's just take one minute here. The Mediterranean diet, as you recall, is high in fruit. It is high in legumes, beans and lentils, green leafy vegetables, and fish, and in the Mediterranean diet we recommend getting rid of that saturated fat, like beef, pork, and lamb, and also limiting saturated fats like butter and cream. The Mediterranean diet also uses the good source of oil, which is olive oil. Of the 10,094 people followed, there were 480 cases of depression and what they found was that the more fruits, nuts, legumes, and mono unsaturated fats consumed the less depression.

Finally, there appears to be a link between depression and bipolar disorder to the high glycemic index diet. We reviewed this diet. This is a diet high in white stuff, white sugar, white flour, so a high glycemic index diet was studied in 691 women. Of these 691 women, 23 were diagnosed with bipolar disorder and what they concluded in the *Journal of Affective Disorders*, which was published in 2011, that bipolar disorder was linked to the high glycemic index diet. Said another way, those women who ate a diet that was high in simple sugar, simple carbohydrates had the higher incidence of bipolar disorder. These four studies clearly demonstrate that a diet of low glycemic foods, whole grains, and omega-3 fatty acids is associated with a lower rate of depression and bipolar disorder—again taking us to the concept that food is medicine.

There is another issue that we need to consider when looking at the role of nutrition and mental well-being. Remember we talked about food sensitivity—and saw how it causes a number of symptoms. These can be gas and bloating, arthritis, joint pains, skin rashes, even mood changes. All of these have been linked to food sensitivity. But, food sensitivity has also been implicated in neurologic disorders of unknown cause.

For example, gluten sensitivity is known in neurology to cause neurologic problems, particularly seizures in people who otherwise had no medical problems. I have to share a personal story. I have a dear friend who called me one day about her 17-year-old daughter and she said that Danika was at school and she started to have a seizure. Well the girl fell and cut her face and all of that was traumatic enough, but she continued to have seizures. She went to the best that Western medicine has to offer. She was flown from neurologist to neurologist. She was on three medications and still she was having seizures. Now this was not a young woman who had had seizures her entire life.

I called up a dear friend of mine who is a holistic integrative neurologist. I said you have to help me out with this girl. The first thing he said was, "Take her off of gluten." He did not even say to do any fancy blood tests or anything like that. Well the end of the story is a happy one. Three years later off of gluten Danika has no more seizures. According to a study published in *Lancet* in 1996, gluten sensitivity is a contributing factor in schizophrenia, bipolar disorder, and anxiety.

We have discussed macronutrition, the proteins, the fats, the foods that we eat, how these are linked to mental well-being and we concluded that the high glycemic index diet is not the way to go; that the Mediterranean diet is evidence-based. What about micronutrients? Things like vitamins and minerals, they appear to be equally as important. Now back to my favorite one, magnesium.

Magnesium deficiency, as we have already seen, is widespread. By now you remember where your magnesium comes from; the greatest source is your green, leafy vegetables. The Horland Health Study evaluated the link between diet and depression in over 5000 people and what they concluded was this: An inverse correlation was found between magnesium intake in the diet and depression scores. In other words the lower the magnesium intake the more likely to be depressed.

Well we have other micronutrients and these micronutrients include things like vitamin D. We have talked about vitamin D before and we pointed out its importance, perhaps, in recurrent breast cancer. We talked about its value in bone health. Vitamin D is really not even a vitamin. It is a hormone. It affects so many different mechanisms and systems in our body.

The brain has vitamin D receptors. A 2005 study showed that low levels of serum 25-hydroxy vitamin D are significantly associated with a higher depression score.

In a second study comparing vitamin D levels in a control group versus a psychiatric population, the psychiatric patients were found to have significantly lower levels of vitamin D. There appears to be this connection between the micronutrients, the vitamins, and mental well-being. Let's take a little look at some more evidence.

What happens if we replace vitamin D? Well a randomized controlled trial did just that. They gave people 20 to 40,000 international units of vitamin D per week and they did this for one year. Then they assessed something called their Beck Depression scores. What they found was there was significant improvement in these scores in those people who received the vitamin D. Now to me, this seems like a simple intervention. Check a vitamin D level, give vitamin D, give magnesium, eat the right diet. This does not seem very complicated.

There is one more that I have to mention. It is so important and that is folate. Folate is a B vitamin and it is one of the most important vitamins for treating depression. Now folate can be used to treat depression with or without antidepressants. As a matter of fact, there are some physicians, psychiatrists, that will give their patients folate whether their level is low or not. When folate is added to an antidepressant medication like Prozac, research shows that there is an improvement in depression above and beyond the effect of the antidepressant alone.

When I see someone who is depressed, as a holistic integrative physician I do not just say here is the antidepressant, first we look at the diet. We look at how someone is living their lives, the foods they are eating, their relationships. We look at their micronutrients and yes there are blood tests available where you can draw blood and assess all of the vitamin levels, you can assess the antioxidant levels. You can even get a blood test for something called an omega-6, omega-3 index. All of these give us a clue as to where you are with your nutritional health.

But my colleagues who practice holistic integrative psychiatry do not stop here. They use the diet, they use the micronutrients, and they absolutely insist that their patients incorporate some kind of exercise into their life. Exercise increases something called brain derived natriuretic factor. Exercise is actually a treatment for depression. The problem is many depressed people say, "I do not feel like exercising." What we do in this situation is we start low and we go slow.

What do I mean by that? Well you heard me say that I want you to exercise one hour a day, but if somebody is really depressed maybe I can get them out walking committing to 15 or 20 minutes, but as we have said before you have to start somewhere. My colleagues in the world of integrative holistic psychiatry might use some other tools for depression. Some of these are very powerful medicine and yes they can be purchased right off the shelf.

One of these is SAM-e. Now I do not recommend that you all go out and say I am feeling depressed and I am down today and Dr. G. said go get some SAM-e. It is true that SAM-e is a potent antidepressant, but it is one of those supplements that has to really be taken under a physician's guidance. Why? Because the dose has to be taken up slowly, over time. We may start at 200 milligrams and slowly increase it up to maybe 800 milligrams per day. I remember once giving a baby little dose of SAM-e to one of my patients and she called me up about a week later and she said, and these were her words, "Dr. G. I'm high as a kite." She said, "I can't sleep at night, I can't stop moving, I'm all over the place." Well that is one of the side effects of SAM-e. It can actually produce a manic state, so in people that have bipolar disorder, which is a combination of depression and mania, we definitely do not want to give SAM-e even if someone has a family history of bipolar disorder, because you may just have the family history of it and never experienced it yourself to any extreme, but the SAM-e might bring out the manic component. Yes, this is a great antidepressant, but please do not just go and start taking it liberally.

There is a second one that has come up in our lectures already and that one is St. John's Wort. Now I know you have heard about St. John's Wort. This is almost as common an herbal remedy as Prozac and Paxil are pharmaceutical remedies. Well St. John's Wort is a good one. It does work for mild to moderate depression. The research shows in severe depression it may not be as effective. You may want to think about something else in that situation, but in mild to moderate depression, 900 milligrams a day of St. John's Wort is a good option, but you may remember what I said about St. John's Wort in the herbal medicine lecture. Depending on the preparation, it can interact with a list of medications that is this long. It can soup up some medications, like other antidepressants, or it can negate the effects of your medications, like in the case of cyclosporine or digoxin or even a blood thinner, Coumadin. This is one that I want you to be careful with and I really want you to find an integrative holistic physician who can guide you on the right use of these supplements.

Now there is something that you can do that really is about as natural as we can get and that is get out in the sunlight. Get out in the sunshine. We call vitamin D the sunshine vitamin so nothing is better than exercising out in the sunlight for depression. There are some people that live in areas where they do not get a lot of sun, particularly in the winter. Let's take a look at one last natural treatment for depression and that is light therapy. One hundred patients in Canada, with depression in winter, were treated with either Prozac or exposure to light. In this case, they sat in front of a light box for 30 to 60 minutes in the morning. Now you may have heard this expression before, seasonal affective disorder; that is SAD. These are people who feel blue during the winter months and we see this in people who live in places like Seattle and like Canada. What happened to these patients? Remember half got Prozac and half got exposed to light. Depression improved equally in both groups, although those receiving the light had a faster response to that improvement, on average two weeks.

The authors concluded that light therapy is as good as the standard antidepressant approach with fewer side effects and much less overall risk and I have to mention one thing here. If you have no pigment in your eyes, like people who have albinism, you may not want to expose your eyes to light therapy. You also may want to check with your physician or your ophthalmologist because if you have a condition like macular degeneration this may not be the right treatment for you, but if your eyes are okay and particularly if you notice, "Gee my depression comes on in the winter, I just feel blue in the winter," light treatment would be a perfect way to go for you.

Let's just review. Our brain needs a balance of nutrients to maintain a positive mood. We talked about nutrition and we said stick with whole foods and a low glycemic index diet. I want you to replace your missing nutrients like vitamin D and magnesium and I want you to add supplements when needed. But the supplements we talked about, SAM-e and St. John's Wort, you may want to talk to your physician about. Finally, get out in the sunlight and exercise because I want you to let nature be your medicine.

Biofield Therapies

Lecture 17

Biofield therapies, which are also referred to as energy medicine, are very controversial in the world of medicine. Although we do not yet have the technology that is capable of measuring the body's biofield, almost every global healing tradition uses biofield medicine in some form. There is ample evidence that, whatever the underlying mechanisms—many yet to be determined—biofield therapies have a positive impact on health. These treatments, including acupuncture, Tai Chi, Qigong, homeopathy, and Healing Touch, need to be an integral part of Western medicine.

The Healing Power of Touch and Energy

- Biofield medicine, or energy medicine, is also sometimes called vibrational medicine because it is believed that in the living body, each electron, atom, chemical, and molecule has a vibratory frequency—as does our body as a whole. Energy medicine seeks to understand this vibratory energy and to interact with this energy in some way to facilitate healing.

- The healing power of touch and energy dates back to Hippocrates, the Greek physician and father of modern medicine. Equally as wise as Hippocrates, Pythagoras, a Greek philosopher and mathematician, referred to the biofield as a vital energy that could produce cures.

- Many cultures have a name for this vital force, or energy field. In China, it is called Chi; in India, as part of Ayurvedic medicine, it is called Prana. In Japan, it is referred to as Ki, and in Polynesia, it is called Mana.

- According to biofield practitioners, the energy system has three key components: energy centers (chakras), energy tracts (meridians), and the energy field (aura).

- The aura surrounds the entire body, and biofield practitioners believe that when people look at pictures of saints and see halos, it is actually an aura.

- The meridians, or energy tracts, run all along the body—up and down the arms and legs—and these energy tracts are where acupuncturists place their needles.

The Concept of Chakras
- There are seven major chakras, or energy centers, in the body. The first chakra is at the spine's base and is called the root chakra. The second chakra is right below the umbilicus and is called the ton-tien. The third is located at the solar plexus. The fourth is the heart. The fifth is located at the throat. The sixth is in the center of the forehead and is called the third eye. The seventh chakra sits at the crown at the top of the head. There are smaller chakras at every joint in the body and in the hands and feet.

- Biofield practitioners believe that each chakra is connected with a function, which can be physical (as it is for the first chakra), emotional (as it is for the second), or mental (as it is for the third). In addition, each chakra is connected to a body gland.

- The function of the heart chakra for biofield practitioners is the concept of love and forgiveness. When people have illnesses related to the heart chakra, it is usually related to love, loss, and forgiveness.

- The fifth chakra sits at the throat, specifically in the thyroid gland. Because the throat is considered the area of expression, when biofield practitioners see someone with a thyroid problem, they start by asking, "Are you expressing yourself?"

Energy-Based Therapy: Acupuncture

- Over 2,500 years old, acupuncture is a key component of traditional Chinese medicine. Acupuncture is based on important energy concepts—most notably, the concept of yin and yang, which explores the important coexistence and necessary balance of opposites not only in the universe but also within each individual.

- In traditional Chinese medicine, it is believed that Chi circulates through the energy tracts and that illness manifests as the result of a blockage or deficiency in one of the tracts. Acupuncture techniques attempt to maintain the balance and reduce the illness by restoring the flow of the Chi through the manipulation of acupuncture points and meridians.

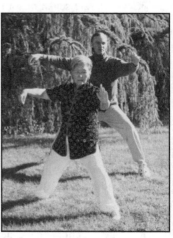

- In 1998, the National Institutes of Health produced a consensus statement endorsing the use of acupuncture for a number of conditions, including elbow tendonitis, plantar fasciitis, muscle spasm, nausea, high blood pressure, infertility, asthma, and addiction.

In addition to acupuncture, homeopathy, and Healing Touch therapies, Tai Chi and Qigong work on the body's energy system.

Energy-Based Therapy: Tai Chi and Qigong

- Other aspects of traditional Chinese medicine are Tai Chi and Qigong, which work on the body's energy system and consist of deep relaxation techniques—including breathing exercises, self-massage, and acupoint stimulation—that involve gentle, fluid movements that are coordinated with the breath to release both physical and emotional stress.

- These exercises leave people feeling relaxed yet revitalized because, according to traditional Chinese medicine, Tai Chi and Qigong exercises promote the flow of energy, or Chi, through the body.

- Tayor Piliae conducted a study to look at whether Tai Chi improved balance, muscle strength, endurance, and flexibility in people with cardiac risk factors and found statistically significant improvement in all of these areas. Tai Chi has also been shown to decrease blood pressure and improve heart rate variability.

Energy-Based Therapy: Homeopathy

- Homeopathy is a natural science that uses plants, minerals, and animal materials in very small doses to stimulate a sick person's disease defenses. "Homos" in Greek means "similar," and "pathos" means "suffering."

- Homeopathy is based on the theory that like cures like; therefore, an energized medicine that mimics a person's symptom will assist in the body's healing process and relieve the symptoms.

- For example, ipecac syrup is used to cause vomiting. It is used in the emergency room if someone has swallowed a poison. However, in the homeopathy world, ipecac is diluted and is used to treat nausea as opposed to induce nausea.

- Homeopathy has wonderful treatments that are safe and that you can use in your home. For example, arnica could be used for any injury or accident. Chamomile is great for children who are cranky—maybe from teeth pain or earaches. Rhus tox is great for sunburns, and calculus can be used for vertigo. All of these are over-the-counter treatments that are standardized and go through FDA approval.

Energy-Based Therapy: Healing Touch

- An energy-based treatment called Healing Touch uses touch to influence the human energy system. As with acupuncture, Healing Touch practitioners believe that disruption in the human energy system is viewed as a blockage of energy flow that needs to be relieved.

- Developed by a nurse named Janet Mentgen, Healing Touch has been extensively endorsed by the American Holistic Nurses Association and is available in many hospitals throughout the United States. Healing Touch helps to relieve fear, decrease pain, and decrease anxiety in patients before and after surgery.

- A study of Marines with post-traumatic stress disorder showed that Healing Touch and guided imagery have a statistically significant reduction in their symptoms.

Questions to Consider

1. What are the three main components of the biofield?

2. Name two global healing traditions that treat the human biofield.

Biofield Therapies
Lecture 17—Transcript

Today we are going to talk about a very controversial field in medicine. Biofield therapies, also called energy medicine, are one of those areas that physicians just can't agree about. Why is it so controversial? I believe it is because we do not yet have a state-of-the-art technology capable of measuring the body's biofield. But as you will see in a few minutes almost every global healing tradition uses biofield medicine in some form. And, as a holistic integrative physician, I have learned from experience that it is really important to keep an open mind.

The best place for me to begin this discussion is with my own story. In the '90s when I was in the cardiac catheterization lab placing stents, I got really sick. I contracted disseminated herpes from a patient. I had never been exposed to the herpes virus. This virus really took me down. We have talked about resiliency, so I bet you can guess that my resiliency in the '90s—with no yoga and meditation in my life (and a crazy on-call schedule did not help the situation)—was low.

It is very unusual for a physician, especially an interventional cardiologist, to miss five or six days of work. On around the sixth day, one of my partners called me and he said, "What is going on? Do you need to be hospitalized?" I told him that I had sores all over my mouth, my glands were out, my neck looked double the size, and immediately he suggested I go into the hospital for IV medication. Now, you can imagine a physician going into your own hospital where you know all the nurses, you know all the staff, not a great situation. I got a second phone call and that was from my nurse, Rounie. She was running the heart program with me at the time, and she said, "I have this technique that I do called Healing Touch. Let me come over and give you a treatment." And I remember exactly what I said to her, I said, "You can do it. As long as it does not involve a lot of needles, I do not mind." She came to my home. I was placed on a massage table and two hours went by. I do not remember what transpired, but I can tell you this: When she finished the treatment, I was able to get up, get dressed, and even the next day I went to work. So I thought to myself: Whatever this treatment is, if it is as good for me as it seems to be, I want this treatment, Healing Touch, available for my patients.

So I went on a journey, and it was a journey to understand everything about biofields or energy medicine. Now, biofield medicine is also called vibrational medicine. Why is it called vibrational medicine? Because it is believed that in the living body, each electron, atom, chemical, and molecule, every organ has a vibratory frequency, as does our body as a whole. So energy medicine seeks to understand this frequency, if you might, this vibratory energy, and to interact with this energy in some way to facilitate healing.

The healing power of touch and energy dates back to Hippocrates, the Greek physician, and father of modern medicine. Hippocrates noted, and I quote, that a "force flowed from peoples' hands." Equally as wise as Hippocrates, Pythagoras in Greece referred to the biofield as, and again, I quote, "Vital energy perceived as a luminous body that could produce cures."

I have to tell you that I really think Pythagoras and Hippocrates were right. And I am not the only one, because many cultures have a name for this vital force or this energy field, and I bet you have heard many of these names. In China it is called Chi; in India, as part of Ayurvedic medicine, it is called Prana. They even have a name for this vital force in Japan, and in Japan it is referred to as Ki. And one of the places I love to travel is Hawaii, and in Polynesia, this vital force is called Mana.

According to biofield practitioners the energy system has three key components: energy centers (which are also called chakras), energy tracts (which are called meridians), and the energy field (which is called the aura).

The aura surrounds the entire body, and biofield practitioners believe that when we look at pictures of saints and we see halos, that that is actually an aura.

The energy tracts run all along the body, up and down the arms, the legs, the entire course of the body. And as you will see in a few minutes, these energy tracts are where acupuncturists place their needles.

Let's spend a minute on the concept of energy centers or chakras. There are seven major chakras in the body. They begin at the base of the spine, so the first chakra is at the spine's base; we call this the root chakra. The second chakra is right below the umbilicus, and what we call the ton-tien. The third is right at the solar plexus. The fourth is the heart. The fifth at the throat, the sixth is in the center of the forehead, and this is called the third eye. And the seventh sits at the crown at the top of the head. There are smaller chakras at every joint in the body, smaller chakras in the hands and in the feet.

How might a biofield practitioner think about this system? I mentioned we have seven chakras, so biofield practitioners believe that each chakra is connected with a function and that function could be physical as it is for the first chakra, emotional, as it is for the second, or mental, as it is for the third. Also, each chakra is connected to a body gland. Let me take my first one for you. My favorite chakra of course, you guessed it, it is the heart. So let's go to the heart chakra.

The function of the heart chakra for biofield practitioners is the concept of love and forgiveness. When people have illnesses related to the heart chakra it usually is related to love, loss, and forgiveness. You know I am a cardiologist, so what organ is sitting right here? The heart. And we use expressions all the time, like, "He died of a broken heart," so it is no surprise to me that this is all connected, the heart chakra, and love. And I have often wondered, does this explain why, when I have couples in my practice that have been together for 60 or 65 years, when one dies, we frequently see the other one die within the next six months, even if they do not have a medical problem? And this has been well proven in the medical literature.

Let me give you a second example. The fifth chakra sits at the throat. Well, there is a gland right there as well that is called the thyroid gland. So, biofield practitioners, when they see someone with a thyroid problem, they would ask a question, "Are you expressing yourself? Because the throat is considered the area of expression." Or put another way, "Are you speaking your truth?"

You can probably tell that I am really fascinated by this, because I learned none of this in medical school. Yet, we see energy-based therapies coming from every global healing tradition. What is amazing to me is they are actually being used today in the west in hospitals and medical settings all over our country. These include techniques like Healing Touch, acupuncture, and Qigong, which come from traditional Chinese medicine. Homeopathy in and of itself is a global healing tradition, and it is a global healing tradition that is based on energy medicine principles. We talked a bit about yoga. Yoga is an integral part of Ayurvedic medicine, and this is the global healing tradition that comes from India. Let's begin with acupuncture.

Acupuncture is well over 2500 years old. As I mentioned, it is a key component of traditional Chinese medicine, but traditional Chinese medicine is more than just acupuncture. Traditional Chinese medicine has a philosophy; it has herbs, and so on. But acupuncture is based on important energy concepts, most notably the concept of yin and yang. I am sure you have heard this. Yin and yang explores the important co-existence and necessary balance of opposites. Not only in the universe, but within each individual. Let me give you an example: light and dark, male and female. So it is about a balance of opposites.

In traditional Chinese medicine it is believed that Chi circulates through the energy tracts, remember, called meridians. What can happen is illness manifests as the result of a blockage or a deficiency in one of these tracts. Acupuncture techniques attempt to maintain balance, to restore the balance back and reduce the illness by restoring the flow of the Chi through the manipulation of acupuncture points and meridians. Sometimes, it is counterintuitive, for example I remember I had back spasm, and I went to an acupuncturist, and my back was hurting so I expected him to put the needles in my back. But he did not; he put the needles in my legs and in my arms. I said to him, "Explain that to me?" He said, "Well the energy tract runs right up your leg, and that is where you have the blockage. This tract," and he pointed down on my leg, "is connected to your back." So this is a very new concept for someone who is practicing Western medicine.

In 1998, the National Institute of Health produced a consensus statement endorsing the use of acupuncture for a number of conditions. They said, "Acupuncture treatment should be considered as adjuvant treatment for pain," all types of pain, elbow tendonitis, plantar fasciitis, one of my favorites: Muscle spasm. That acupuncture could be considered for nausea, for pregnant women, nausea from surgery, nausea from chemotherapy. Should be considered for people that have high blood pressure. People that have infertility, people that have asthma, and people that have addiction.

In my current practice at Scripps, I have two physician colleagues who practice acupuncture, so they are MDs who are formally trained to also be acupuncturists. I think of them as bridge people, we talked about that earlier on. And I have three licensed acupuncturists; I have a nurse who is licensed in acupuncture and two other acupuncturists as well. So I have an office of acupuncturists.

You might be thinking why would a cardiologist have an office of acupuncturists? Let me explain why. As a cardiologist, I teach my patients proper nutrition. We talked a lot about that. And, I teach them, of course, to exercise. But what would they come back and say? They say, "I can't exercise, my back hurts, my knee hurts, my foot hurts." I needed a way to relieve their pain without giving them another drug. Some of you may recall there was a big medicine brouhaha over a drug called Vioxx. When that drug was on the market, we were seeing a lot of issues because if it was not given in the right dose or it was given in too high a dose, it really caused high blood pressure, and other cardiac problems. So that kind of medication is definitely not something I want in one of my heart patients. Also, most of the pain medicine, even if it is Motrin or Aleve or Advil, can irritate the stomach lining, and if you have ulcers or kidney disease, we do not want you on those medicines, so I needed a different option, and for my patients, I chose acupuncture.

Another aspect of traditional Chinese medicine is Tai Chi and Qigong. Tai Chi and Qigong also work on the body's energy system, but differently. They consist of deep relaxation techniques, breathing exercise, self-massage, even acupoint stimulation. You can actually learn the points to help with things like nausea, and you can treat yourself. You may be most familiar with the exercises that we see people doing, even sometimes right out in the parks, these gentle, fluid movements, coordinated with the breath, to release both physical and emotional stress. That is Tai Chi and Qigong.

These exercises leave people feeling relaxed yet revitalized. That is how I feel after meditation. I am relaxed, but I am ready to go. That is a great combination. So how do they do that? Well, according to traditional Chinese medicine, the Tai Chi and Qigong exercises promote the flow of energy through the body. Again, the energy known as Chi.

Let's take a look at two studies on Tai Chi. The first was conducted by Taylor-Piliae. They conducted a study to look at whether Tai Chi improved balance, muscle strength, endurance, and flexibility in people with cardiac risk factors. So, 39 adults participated, they did 60 minutes of Tai Chi class three times a week, and they found this: Statistically significant improvement in balance, muscle strength, endurance, and flexibility at six weeks and at twelve weeks.

Why is that important? It is important because if you have more flexibility and more balance and more muscle strength, there is a very good chance you are not going to fall, and if you do not fall, we do not have to deal with one of those devastating hip fractures that claim people's lives, so Tai Chi is a wonderful exercise for improving muscle strength.

A second study was done in 2004 by Gloria Yeh. Thirty patients were randomized to a Tai Chi group or a non-Tai Chi group. This group of patients had congestive heart failure. They did 12 weeks of Tai Chi or standard care—that is, going to their physician. Patients in the Tai Chi group demonstrated marked improvement in what is called a six-minute walk test. This test is an indicator of heart improvement, of cardiac improvement, no surprise because we just saw that muscles get better, we become more flexible, so many cardiologists today tell their patients, "Go and take a class in Tai Chi." And Tai Chi has also been shown to decrease blood pressure and improve heart rate variability. Remember, we talked about heart rate variability; if the heart rate variability is low, we run a risk of sudden death, so improving heart rate variability is key.

Let's take a look at another global healing tradition, this time homeopathy. Because homeopathy has energy medicine embedded right within it. Homeopathy is a natural science; it uses plants, minerals, and animal materials in very small doses to stimulate a sick person's disease defenses.

The best way to think about it is it works like a vaccine. If I give you a low dose of something, hopefully I am not going to make you sick, like most vaccines do not make you sick, but I am going to stimulate your body's response in case you get exposed to that virus, for example. Well, homos in Greek means similar, and pathos means suffering. Homeopathy is based on the theory that like cures like, therefore, an energized medicine that mimics a person's symptom will assist in the body's healing process. It will relieve the symptoms. Let me give you an example: Ipecac syrup is used to cause vomiting. It is used in the emergency room if someone has swallowed a poison. But, in the homeopathy world, ipecac is diluted so many times that when it is given, it is actually given for nausea. It actually is used to treat nausea as opposed to induce nausea. Again, think of the vaccine scenario, it stimulates the body's healing response.

Hippocrates said, "Through the like disease is produced, and through the like disease is cured." Homeopathy is used around the world. It is taught in German medical schools; 25 percent of German physicians use homeopathy. In England, 42 percent of general practitioners refer to homeopaths. In India, they have 125 homeopathic medical schools.

In 1991 the *British Medical Journal* published a meta-analysis of 107 controlled trials using homeopathy, and concluded this: 81 were effective, 24 were ineffective, and two were inconclusive. I think 81 effective trials are worth looking at. But do not worry; I am not going to tell you anything about 81 trials. But what I think you should think about is having some homeopathy in your home. Homeopathy has wonderful treatments that are safe, that you can use and you can even use them on children. Let's just look at a few.

Let's take arnica, for example. Arnica could be used for any injury, any accident. Arnica is a good one to have. I like chamomile; this is great for children. Sounds like chamomile, right? Relaxing tea? Well, chamomile is wonderful for children who are a little cranky, maybe from teeth pain, or earaches. Rhus tox is wonderful for sunburns. And there is even a good homeopathic remedy called calculus, for vertigo. All of these are over-the-counter, yet they are all standardized and they go through FDA approval. I love to have a few homeopathic remedies available at home, and you might want to do that, too.

Let's talk now about a treatment that I have been using at Scripps for many, many years. At Scripps, we have been doing an energy-based treatment called Healing Touch since 1993. Healing Touch uses touch to influence the human energy system. That is the treatment that was done on me. This is the field that surrounds the body. As with acupuncture, Healing Touch practitioners believe that disruption in the human energy system is viewed as a blockage of energy flow. It is this blockage that needs to be relieved, because it can produce disease or we can even get a blockage that results from disease. Healing Touch was developed by a nurse, Janet Mentgen, and has been extensively endorsed by the American Holistic Nurses Association. Since 1993 we have been teaching nurses at Scripps Healing Touch, and this is available in many hospitals throughout the country. In our hospital we have a Healing Touch practitioner right on the floor. Why? Because people in the hospital have a lot of pain, they have a lot of anxiety, they have a lot of fear, and Healing Touch is a great technique to help to relieve fear, decrease pain, and decrease anxiety. We looked at Healing Touch in 200 patients before and after bypass surgery, and we found that pre-surgery, we were able to decrease a patient's anxiety. Post-surgery, we were able to decrease anxiety. People are worried about what is going to happen to them when they go home. We were also able to show that post-surgery, we were able to decrease pain.

More recently in 2010, we conducted a study with the Camp Pendleton Marines, active Marines with a diagnosis of Post Traumatic Stress Disorder. These Marines were randomized to a control group or a group that received Healing Touch and guided imagery. I can't give you the details of all this data because it is in press, but I will tell you this: Those Marines that were randomized to Healing Touch and guided imagery had a statistically significant reduction in their Post Traumatic Stress Disorder symptoms. The military is looking at these techniques to help returning soldiers.

I want you to remember that everything can be assessed energetically. Have you ever walked into a room and thought oh, I do not want to be here, this place feels uncomfortable. You were actually sensing what we would call the energy of the place. Or have you ever been around a person that you say, "I really like your energy," well what do you mean by that?

At the top of the lecture I noted that biofield therapies are controversial, in large because we do not have some big machine that we can put people into and measure that biofield. But it is my personal hope that these technologies will be developed in the future. In the meantime, I believe we have ample evidence that whatever the underlying mechanisms, many yet to be determined, biofield therapies have a positive impact on health. I have seen that positive impact in my practice and my own life. And that is why I am persuaded that these treatments need to be an integral part of our Western medicine toolbox.

In the end, I invite you to reach your own conclusions. Take a look at the research on acupuncture, Tai Chi, homeopathy, and Healing Touch. And, if you are ready, you might even take a Tai Chi class, or consider acupuncture for some of the conditions we have talked about. As I have learned, experience is often the best evidence you can have.

The Power of Love
Lecture 18

People have all types of relationships in their lives that show them who they are. These relationships begin as children with their parents, and as adults, people have work partners, colleagues, and friends. In this lecture, you will begin to explore the notion of whether relationships impact health. You will look at relationships with parents, spouses and partners, and even larger social networks to conclude that healthy relationships, social connections—to family, friends, and spiritual communities—and optimism are essential ingredients to good health.

Relationships with Parents

- The Harvard Mastery of Stress Study, in which 126 male Harvard students were studied for 35 years, looked at whether parental relationships had an effect on disease in midlife. Participants who identified their relationships with their parents as strained had a 100 percent incidence of significant health risk—including coronary disease, cancer, hypertension, ulcers, and alcohol abuse—35 years later. Amazingly, participants whose relationships with their parents were warm and close cut this risk from 100 percent to 47 percent.

- Researchers reasoned that the results can be explained because we learn everything from our parents, including nutrition, exercise habits, coping styles, and conflict resolution. Our parents also give us our spiritual values and spiritual practices.

- A study conducted over 50 years at Johns Hopkins University concluded that cancer rates correlated closely with the degree of closeness to a parent.

- The Adverse Childhood Experiences (ACE) Study, which was conducted by a physician named Vincent Felitti on adverse childhood events, found that the more trauma a child faces—such as fighting in the home, hitting among parents, parents being in jail, and sexual abuse—the higher the risk of major illness in midlife and the higher the risk of drug and alcohol abuse.

Relationships with Spouses and Partners

- In a study that was reported in *The American Journal of Medicine*, about 10,000 men who were identified with three or more cardiac risk factors were asked about how they perceived their wife's love. Five years later, those who had responded that their wife showed them love had a 50 percent lower rate of angina—the manifestation of coronary artery disease—onset than those who had responded that their wife did not show them love.

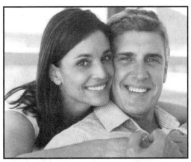

Studies have shown that people who have a close connection with another person often have much less stress.

- In 1992, a study that was reported in the *Journal of the American Medical Association* asked 1,400 men and women whose actual coronary anatomy was known whether they were married or had a confidant. People who were not married and had no close confidant had three times the death rate of the other groups over five years. If people have a close connection with someone, they often have much less stress.

- A study of over 9,000 British civil servants that looked at the relationship between unhappy marriages and heart disease was conducted over a period of 12 years. Researchers concluded that unhappy marriages (which often contain a great deal of stress) led to 34 percent more coronary events—regardless of variables such as gender and social status.

- There are many factors that contribute to a good relationship versus a bad one, including being optimistic. A group of couples was studied over a two-year period, and researchers found that optimism is clearly linked to happier and more satisfied romantic relationships. They concluded that this was due to greater cooperative problem solving.

- Optimists see the good in their partner; they are not focusing on the little things that sometimes can become annoying. Research shows that optimists have a 55 percent lower risk of death from all causes and a 23 percent lower risk of cardiovascular death.

The Impact of Social Networks on Health

- In the 1950s and 1960s, epidemiologists discovered that a group of Italians that had moved from a small town in Italy to Roseto, Pennsylvania, were not having heart attacks at the same rate as people found in the surrounding communities. However, those family members who moved away from Roseto developed heart disease at the same rate as whatever community they moved to.

- Epidemiologists attributed the protection from heart disease to the social network—the household and the community—and called this phenomenon the Roseto effect. It was common for households in Roseto to contain three generations, and there was a high degree of religiosity and traditional family values. After the 1970s, when children began to move away, there was a breakdown of these multigenerational households and an increase in heart attack prevalence, possibly as a result of increased stress.

- A researcher named Nancy Frasure-Smith conducted a study that looked at social support and depression. She studied 880 people who had already had a heart attack and found that even in people who were severely depressed, the effect of the depression on their cardiac death rates was negated if they felt a good sense of social support.

- The Alameda County Study was a 17-year study of 7,000 men and women that found that people who lack social contact—those who do not have friends, relatives, or social groups—had a 3.1-fold higher death rate. This study controlled for such variables as age, sex, smoking, eating, and alcohol.

- In a study that was conducted in 1997, 276 healthy people were asked to have the rhinovirus placed in their nose, and those with the least number of social connections were four times more likely to get the cold virus infection.

- A study of over 700 older adults looked at an important spiritual principle—that it is better to give than to receive—by pairing the adults with younger children to read, color, or have some sort of interaction. The researchers found that those who gave love and support to others had significantly fewer health issues.

- David Speigel conducted a study in which he created a support group to help women adjust to their diagnosis of breast cancer. The women with breast cancer were asked to participate in a 90-minute group session once a week for one year. The women in the support group showed less depression, anger, and anxiety, but they also lived twice as long as women in the control group.

- A similar study was done that involved patients with melanoma, a very malignant form of skin cancer. Patients were randomized to six weeks of group support versus a control and were studied for five years. Researchers found 13 recurrences of melanoma in the control group versus seven in the group that went to group support and 10 deaths in the control group versus only three in the support group.

Questions to Consider

1. How are unhappy relationships linked to coronary disease?

2. Can the impact of depression on health be negated by social connection?

The Power of Love
Lecture 18—Transcript

My grandmother used to say, "Show me who your friends are, and I will show you who you are." We have all types of relationships in our life. These relationships start as children with our parents, and as adults we have work partners, colleagues, and friends. I agree with my grandmother's wisdom that relationships show us who we are. As a physician, I can't help but wonder, do relationships impact health?

Today, we will begin to explore that very question. We will look at relationships, relationships with our parents, spouse and partner, and even larger social networks.

Let's start at the beginning and look at our first relationship, the relationship with our parents. Can that relationship impact our health?

An incredible study was conducted called "The Harvard Mastery of Stress Study." 126 male Harvard students were studied for 35 years. The point of the study was to look at whether or not parental relationships had any effect at all on disease 35 years later in midlife. They asked these participants four questions: Describe your relationship with your mom and with your dad, and was it very close, was it warm and friendly, was it tolerant, or was it strained and cold? Well, I find what they found totally amazing. If you identified your relationship with your parents as strained, there was a 100 percent incidence of significant health risk 35 years later. This included things like coronary disease, cancer, hypertension, ulcers, even alcohol abuse. Now, what if your relationship was warm and close? You cut this risk from 100 percent to 47 percent. That is an amazing difference.

I think even the researchers were amazed at what they found. They tried to explain these results, and this is what they concluded. Actually, their conclusions make a lot of sense to me. They said, "What do we learn from our parents?" Basically we learn everything. We learn how to eat from our parents. We learn our exercise habits from our parents. Our coping styles frequently come from our parents. If you show me someone who is angry, and tries to resolve conflict by anger, there is a good chance that that person learned that style from their parents. On a deeper level, our parents give us our spiritual values and our spiritual practices. They teach us what is important in life.

A second study was conducted at Johns Hopkins, and followed in this case for 50 years. The Johns Hopkins study took over 1000 medical students, and they looked at closeness to parents. What they concluded 50 years later was that cancer rates correlated closely with the degree of closeness to a parent.

I have to tell you about one of my colleagues. I have a friend and fellow physician named Vince Feletti who is living in San Diego, and has conducted years of research on what is called adverse childhood events. What made him do this was that he started to notice that when people had addictions later in life, they seemed to come from troubled childhood families, so this sent him on a quest where he studied over 18,000 people. His study is called "The ACE Study" or "Adverse Childhood Events Study." What the research shows is the more trauma a child faces such as fighting in the home, hitting among parents, parents being in jail, sexual abuse, the higher the risk of major illness in midlife, but also a much higher risk of drug and alcohol abuse.

So what do we do? Are we stuck if we had less than optimal relationships with our parents? No, of course not. We are not stuck; we all need to embrace our past. We do not want to become victims of our past, and as you will see, later on, forgiveness and acceptance is the key.

So how we grow up can affect illness 35 and 50 years later. What else can affect our health? Well let's take a look at relationships with our spouse and partner. What impact do these have?

An interesting study was reported in *The American Journal of Medicine*. This was a great question. Some 10,000 men who were already identified with three or more cardiac risk factors asked, "Does your wife show you love?" What a great question. It is their perception of love. And then these guys were followed for five years and what they found was this: Those who answered yes, their wife showed them love, had a 50 percent lower rate of chest discomfort, angina, actually the manifestation of coronary artery disease, a 50 percent lower rate of anginal onset than those who answered no. So I know a lot of you are turning to your wife right now and saying, "Show me love." And it is an important question.

Another interesting question reported in *The Journal of the American Medical Association* in 1992 asked: Are you married or do you have a confidant? And this question was asked of 1400 men and women. So these men and women had a cardiac catheterization, so their actual coronary anatomy was known. The variables were, "Are you married?" or "Do you have someone you can confide in?" This is what they found: People who were not married and had no close confidant had three times the death rate of the other groups over five years. Are you connected? That is what this study is saying. Do you have someone that you can talk to, that you can confide in, a confidant? That could be your spouse or maybe it is not your spouse, someone that you can tell some of your deepest, darkest concerns to. That is what this study tells me, because if we have that kind of connection, there is a pretty good chance we have a lot less stress.

Let's take a look at another marriage study. This study was conducted in Britain, and it looked at the relationship between unhealthy marriages or unhappy marriages and heart disease. They studied over 9000 British civil servants. In this study, they had 6000 men and about 2800 women. They were also followed a long time, for 12 years. This is what they concluded: Unhappy marriages led to 34 percent more coronary events regardless of things like gender and social status. Just being in an unhappy marriage. Now, I do not have to tell you, it makes total sense. We talked already about stress, the stress hormones, and the impact of stress on our heart.

Now, of course there are many facts that contribute to a good relationship versus a poor relationship. There are many variables. Let's take a look at one of them. Does being optimistic in a relationship make a difference? One group of couples was studied over a two-year period, and the researchers found that optimism is clearly linked to happier and more satisfied romantic relationships. They concluded that this was due to greater cooperative problem solving. Another study reported in the *Journal of Personality and Social Psychology* in 2006 demonstrated that optimistic couples resolve conflict faster, see the other as supportive, and live up to the other's ideals and expectations. So, to me, this gets back to what we previously discussed; the optimists are positive. I think it is about the power of being positive; their glass is half full. They see the good in their partner; they are not focusing on those little things that sometimes can become annoying. It is all a matter of where we put our focus, do we see the big picture, or do we just see the toothpaste in the bathroom sink?

Could that explain why optimists live longer? Because they do, 999 men and women were followed over nine years, and they were divided into four groups, and the groups assessed their level of optimism. Optimists had a 55 percent lower risk of death from all causes, and a 23 percent lower risk of cardiovascular death. So clearly, optimism is good for our relationships but it is also good for our health.

So up to this point we have been focusing on intimate relationships, our relationship with our parents, and our relationship with our partners. Now let's broaden the conversation a little bit. Let's take a look at the impact of our social networks on our health.

A wonderful spiritual teacher named Satchidananda had this to say, "The I in illness is isolation. The W E in wellness is we." Well, is there research out there to support Satchidananda's claim?

Let's go to Roseto, Pennsylvania. I want to talk for a few minutes on this amazing study, the Roseto study. Italians moved from a little town in Italy to Pennsylvania and they kept immigrating over the course of time. The town of Roseto attracted the epidemiologists. They said: Why is it that in this one little town, people are not having heart attacks? They are smoking, they have diabetes, and they have cholesterol. So the epidemiologists decided they were going to go into Roseto and take a look at things like soil, air, water, they really wanted to understand why they were not having heart attacks at the same rate as all of the surrounding communities. What was so special about Roseto?

Well, as they started to look at the community, they realized it had nothing to do with the water, the air, the food, it could not be explained by any of those things. They also knew years later that those family members that picked up and moved from Roseto developed heart disease at the same rate as whatever community they were in. So they concluded this: They called it the Roseto Effect, and they said it was about the household and the community. There were three-generation households in Roseto. Grandma was in the house with parents and children. This was very common. There was a high degree of religiosity, traditional values; families ate together. They attributed the protection from heart disease to the social network. After the 1970s children began to move away, there was a breakdown of these multigenerational households; with the increased mobility the heart attack prevalence was the same as the surrounding communities. The authors concluded the golden age of Roseto was over.

Now, I grew up in one of those families. My grandmother was in the house cooking all day, aunts were around, parents were around; it was a big community. It was a tribe, if you might. This is common, extended families in Italian households, and it has a profound effect on health. Why do I think so? Because there is less stress.

A researcher named Nancy Frasure-Smith also did an interesting study looking at social support, and she studied depression. She took 880 people who had already had a heart attack. Now, we know that depression is an independent risk factor for heart disease. Depressed people do not say, "Oh, I am going to eat Dr. Guarneri's Brussels sprouts and broccoli and go and exercise." There is a good chance if you are depressed you might say, "I am not exercising today, and this donut is making me feel really good." So depression is a big concern for me in my practice. She looked at Beck depression scales, and she looked at how depressed people were, but she did something else, she looked at whether or not they felt socially supported, whether they had community, family around them. This is what she found: She found that even in people who were severely depressed, the effect of the depression on their heart, on their cardiac death rates was negated if they felt a good sense of social support. To me, that is powerful, powerful medicine.

One more study, this is the Alameda County Study, a 17-year study of 7000 men and women. Those who lack social contact, what I say being home alone, people who do not have friends, relatives, churches, social groups, anything, had a 3.1-fold higher death rate, and in this study, they controlled for everything else, age, sex, smoking, eating, alcohol, all those other things that you may be thinking about. What they concluded is that it was about social connection.

One of my favorite studies appeared in *JAMA* in 1997, where 276 healthy people were asked to have the rhinovirus placed in their nose. I do not know about you, but I don't know that I would have volunteered for this study. What they were looking at was really resiliency. We talked about the soil and being resilient. So they looked at social connections, 12 different types of relationships, things we have been talking about, parents, childhood, groups, connection. Everyone had the virus inserted in their nose, and no surprise, those with the least number of social connections were four times more likely to get the cold virus infection.

So if relationships are so important, can creating social connection be a treatment? I remember when we did the Ornish research in the 1990s. We had something called the cohort effect. Now, cohort means band of warriors, and we were bringing groups of really sick patients, 10 or 15 or 20 at a time. These people had bad coronary disease, they were depressed, they were diabetic, they were overweight, they had all of these medical problems. And what we noticed almost immediately was that when they came into the cardiac rehab groups together, they came to life. They now had 20 new friends, people they can exercise with, they would start calling each other at home, they became socially connected, they prepared meals together. We conducted this research in the '90s. I still have patients from that original study—now this is 15 years later—that are getting together to have meals, to walk, and just to talk about life. So to me, it was so much more important than what their cholesterol level was. Yes, I was concerned about cholesterol and you know I was concerned about blood pressure, but it was this entity, if you might, that we called the cohort effect, just being together, remembering the W E in wellness.

There is one other study that I really liked a lot, and it is a study that looked at an important spiritual principle, and that principle is it is better to give than receive. This was a study of over 700 older adults. If you look in almost any culture, you will usually find the grandparent paired with the youngest. This is normal. So what this study looked at was what if we took older adults and paired them with younger children? Whether it is to read, to color, to do some sort of interaction. This is what they found: Those who gave love and support to others had significantly fewer health issues.

If it is so important to have a social network, can we use this concept of social network, like I did in my heart program, to actually be a treatment for disease? Can it impact the course of a chronic disease? I think the answer is yes, and let's take a look at some research.

David Speigel has done some very interesting research in women with breast cancer. He conducted a study in which he created a support group to help women adjust to their diagnosis of breast cancer. What he was looking for was, could he decrease their depression, their anxiety, and their stress? The women with breast cancer were asked to participate in a 90-minute group session once a week for one year. Well, he got his outcome. Women in the support group showed less depression, less anger, less anxiety. But this is what shocked everyone: The women in the support groups lived twice as long, 18 months compared to nine months in the control group. And an additional study was done that was very similar, looking at melanoma. Patients with a very malignant form of skin cancer, melanoma, were randomized to six weeks of group support versus a control. They were studied for five years; that is a long time. They found 13 recurrences of melanoma in the control group versus seven in the group that went to group support. That is almost half the amount. Take a look at the deaths, 10 deaths in the control groups versus only three with group support.

So as I have seen with my patients, one of the key ingredients to health is connection, social connection, connection to family, connection to friends, and as you will see in a later lecture, connection to spiritual community.

I still have the cohort effect going on at my cardiac rehab program. One of my greatest joys is when someone comes to see me in my office and it is very clear that they are home alone and isolated, and they are living with the fear of coronary artery disease. And when I convince them to come into our lifestyle change program, which means they get to come and be at our center three times a week, invariably these people tell me, "This has changed my life." And it is not about their blood pressure or cholesterol; it is about their new connections, their social network, and their friends.

We have talked about the health impact of relationships through every stage of life. We concluded that healthy relationships, social connection, and optimism are essential ingredients to good health. As we have said in previous lectures, through what lens do you see? And as we discussed earlier Satchidananda said the W E in wellness is indeed, we.

Spirituality in Health
Lecture 19

As Florence Nightingale said, "The needs of the spirit are as crucial to health as those individual organs which make up the body." In this lecture, you will explore what research has revealed about the relationship between spirituality and health. To treat the whole person—body, mind, emotions, and spirit—and to guide patients to find inner peace, integrative holistic medicine physicians use such techniques as guided imagery, meditation, yoga, breathing techniques, repetitive prayer, mantras, and Healing Touch.

The Connection between Spirituality and Health

- Spirituality is a sense of connection with the source of ultimate meaning. Frequently, spirituality includes connection with oneself, with others, with nature, or with a higher power. This connection helps an individual make sense of his or her life.

- For many people, spirituality is truly a quest for meaning and wholeness. Whether we want to admit it or not, science cannot answer all the questions; the human heart has a hidden want that science cannot supply.

- We can think of religion as a way of life. Religion includes a community and connection to others, has a philosophy, and is frequently associated with service. Religion also has traditions, practices, and rituals.

- Spirituality may or may not involve formal religion, but spirituality is almost always included in religious practices.

- In 2001, the Mayo Clinic reported that 90 percent of people believe in a higher being, 94 percent of people regard their spiritual and physical health as equally important, and 96 percent of family practice physicians believe that spiritual well-being is a factor in health. More and more research shows a strong connection between spirituality and health.

- In 2000, a meta-analysis of 42 studies involving nearly 126,000 people was published in the *Journal of Health Psychology* that found that highly religious people had 29 percent higher odds of survival compared with less religious people. The authors were unable to attribute this finding to any confounding variables—or even to publication bias.

- Another study that looked at religion and mortality followed 5,286 adults for 28 years and was published in the *American Journal of Public Health*. Those who attended religious services at least once per week had a 23 percent reduction in their mortality. This study adjusted for variables such as age, sex, ethnicity, education, body mass index, and health practices.

- Data from the Mayo Clinic show that religious people have lower blood pressure, are more likely to comply with their medications, are more likely to exercise more often and eat healthier foods, and even have healthier habits—including giving up cigarettes and alcohol. In addition, they are more likely to use preventative health services. They also found that religious individuals are more accepting of death. They have less depression and anxiety, and they are less likely to abuse drugs. The research even showed that they were less likely to commit suicide.

- A 23-year prospective study that was conducted with 10,059 male Israeli civil servants found that Orthodox Jewish men had a 20 percent decreased risk of a fatal heart attack or heart disease when compared with nonreligious men. The researchers that conducted this study adjusted for age, blood pressure, cholesterol, smoking, diabetes, and mass index—all the baseline risks.

- Another study that was conducted in Israel demonstrated that secular Jews had a higher chance of having a first heart attack when compared with Orthodox Jews. As in the first study, age, ethnicity, education, smoking, and physical exercise were all controlled for, so the authors concluded that there was something about the connection to religion and spirituality that led to health.

- People who are religious or spiritual experience health advantages partly because they have a very strong social support network. People who are spiritual also tend to have increased hope, more contentment, and more peace, and they also tend to be more optimistic. The combination of all of these factors results in the negation of the stress hormones.

- It is possible that people who are spiritual or religious have less medical problems because they turn their problems over to a higher power. When they do that, they remove the burden from themselves.

Addressing Depression and Hopelessness

- Depression has a 40 percent higher coronary artery disease rate and a 60 percent higher death rate. Depression is often found in conjunction with hopelessness.

- People who come into a hospital and are depressed and feeling hopeless—especially people who already have documented coronary artery disease—are less likely to do well with surgery. They have more post-surgical complications, including a two-fold increase risk in outpatient mortality and a five-fold increase in death after a first heart attack.

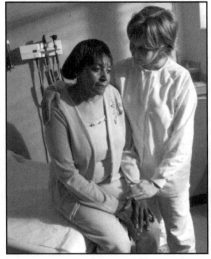

Depression materializes in people who lose the peace and rhythm of life and who lack meaning and purpose in life.

- When people feel hopeless and give up, they are less likely to comply with those things that will improve their heart rate variability and make them healthy. If someone is feeling hopeless, telling them to exercise and eat well is probably not going to work.

- When someone goes through the trauma of a big surgery, they appear to be terrified and shocked afterward. When the physician tries to talk to these patients, they often blindly stare back at them. In other words, the person who had the surgery is simply not there. They are experiencing emotional trauma.

- In these situations, Native Americans might say, "Call your spirit back." The act of calling your spirit back to you involves reconnecting with what is important in your life. It is about finding hope, establishing community, changing your perspective on any health challenges, and ultimately, finding inner peace.

- In addition to guided imagery, meditation, yoga, breathing techniques, repetitive prayer, mantras, and Healing Touch, there are some other equally important aspects of spirituality that integrative holistic medicine physicians use to address depression and hopelessness—including practicing forgiveness and gratitude and experiencing the power of positive thinking. When all of these techniques are combined, physicians are not just healing the physical body—they are integrating body, mind, emotions, and spirit. The physical, mental, and emotional aspects of healing cannot be separated.

Questions to Consider

1. What is the difference between spirituality and religion?

2. What are two ways in which a spiritual crisis may present itself?

Spirituality in Health
Lecture 19—Transcript

Welcome back. Florence Nightingale had this to say, "The needs of the spirit are as crucial to health as those individual organs which make up the body." Do we have science to back up Florence Nightingale's claim? In this lecture, we will explore what research has revealed about the relationship between spirituality and health.

There are many definitions for spirituality. One is spirituality is a sense of connection with the source of ultimate meaning. Frequently, spirituality includes connection with oneself, with others, with nature, or a higher power. This connection helps an individual make sense of their life.

Why is there so much interest in spirituality? For many people, it is truly a quest for meaning and for wholeness. Whether we want to admit it or not, science cannot answer all the questions. The human heart has a hidden want which science can't supply. This quote from Sir William Osler sums it up: "A hidden want, or a hidden desire for which we may not have an answer."

Benjamin Rush found that hidden want in religion. He said, "A religion of some kind is as essential to the mind as air is to respiration."

We can think of religion as a way of life. And it includes community and connection to others. Religion includes a philosophy, and it is frequently associated with service. Religion also has traditions, practices, and rituals.

In my practice, I always ask people about their spiritual practices, whether they consider themselves religious or spiritual. And many people today tell me they consider themselves spiritual. So spirituality may or may not involve formal religion, but it is almost always included in religious practices.

Why is this even important in medicine? And why would a cardiologist even be talking about it? Well, the Mayo Clinic in 2001 reported the following statistics: 90 percent of people believe in a higher being. Ninety-four percent of people regard their spiritual and physical health as equally important.

And even 96 percent of family practice physicians believe that spiritual well being is a factor in health.

With numbers like these, it is not surprising that more and more research is showing a strong connection between spirituality and health. Let's take a look at some of that research.

A meta-analysis was published in the year 2000 in the *Journal of Health Psychology*. This meta-analysis reviewed 42 studies, nearly 126,000 people, and what they found was that highly religious people had 29 percent higher odds of survival compared with less religious people. The authors were unable to attribute this finding to any confounding variables, or even to publication bias. A second study to look at religion and mortality was published in the *American Journal of Public Health*; 5286 adults were followed for 28 years. Those who attended religious services at least once per week had a 23 percent reduction in their mortality. This study also adjusted for things like age, sex, ethnicity, education, and so on. Even physical parameters like body mass index, health practices, and still there was a 23 percent reduction in mortality in those who attended religious services.

Further data from the Mayo Clinic may have the answer to why spiritually active people live longer. Their data shows that religious attenders have lower blood pressure, are more likely to comply with their medications, are definitely more likely to exercise more, eat healthier foods, and even have healthier habits. They are more likely to give up cigarettes and alcohol. In addition, they are more likely to use preventative health services. They also found that religious individuals are more accepting of death. They have less depression and anxiety, and they are less likely to abuse drugs. The research even showed they were less likely to commit suicide.

Now, I am fascinated by this, and whenever I think about religion and health, and spirituality and health, I have to think about my patients Lillian and George. Let me describe Lillian and George to you: Lillian is 95 and George is 97. They have been together for over 60-some-odd years. They are tall, they are thin, they can bend down and pick things up quickly, they have no physical limitations that I can see. They have been vegan their entire life. They are very careful to tell me, "Dr. G., we walk 2.5 miles a day, exactly

2.5 miles a day." George is a minister. He teaches Bible study. Lillian goes with George every week to the Bible study class. She has been doing this for over 60 years. So they are very connected, they are connected to their spiritual community; they are connected to each other. So I asked my cardiac residents, what is it that is helping George and Lillian to be doing so well at 95 and 97? Well, George and Lillian are members of the Seventh Day Adventist community, and as part of their religion, health is considered a key component. Lillian once said to me, "Health is being closer to God." But research is showing similar health benefits across a wide range of religious traditions. Let's take a look at one.

A 23-year prospective study was conducted in 10,059 male Israeli civil servants. What they found was that Orthodox Jewish men had a 20 percent decreased risk of a fatal heart attack or heart disease when compared with non-religious men. They looked at everything, they adjusted for age and blood pressure and cholesterol and smoking and diabetes, how big they were, mass index, all the baseline risks, and still at the end of the day, over 10,000 people studied, a 20 percent decrease in fatal cardiac events in those people that were Orthodox and had strong religious values.

Another study also conducted in Israel, demonstrated that secular Jews had a higher chance of having a first heart attack when compared with Orthodox Jews. As in the first study, everything was controlled for, age ethnicity, education, smoking, physical exercise, the authors had to conclude at the end of the day that there was something about the connection to religion and spirituality that led to health.

I bet some of you had a similar experience to what I have had in my life, where you are working longer and harder, and harder and longer, and work stops becoming a joy. I love my patients; I can certainly live without the administration. But for me as a physician, I know that the day I began to see my work as service, I no longer felt like it was work. When my spiritual life started to open, I changed my whole perspective on what I do every day. The research shows that physicians with a spiritual life are 25 percent happier. I know that this is true for me.

So at the end of the day, what do we attribute this to? What do we really think it is about? Why do we see these health advantages in people who are religious, people who are spiritual? What advantage do they have? I tell you what I think it comes down to: It comes down to a very strong social support network. I know when my patients have surgery, if they are a part of a spiritual community, or a religious group, it really does not matter, they have a whole team mobilizing around them, not only to take care of them, but to support their spouse, their children, whatever they need. I remember one of my patients saying, "When my husband had his bypass, I did not have to cook for a month, because my community," which she called her tribe, "brought new food every single day." So I think that is important. People who are spiritual also tend to have increased hope, more contentment, more peace in their life, and they also tend to be more optimistic. So think about this combination, stronger social support, more love, more hope, more contentment, more optimism. You know the effect this is going to have on the stress hormones. They are going to be negated. I think that is why people who are spiritual and religious have less medical problems. I think, quite frankly, they turn their problems over to a higher power. And when you can do that, you take the burden off of you.

There is a Cheyenne proverb that says, "When you lose the rhythm of the drumbeat of God, you are lost from the peace and rhythm of life." That is truly important, the peace and rhythm of life. Now you may not think, as a cardiologist, I see this in my practice, but I see it every day, only it comes in under different names. It comes in to my practice as depression. It comes in as hopelessness. I see it as isolation. My patients frequently describe it as stress, or they will say to me, "I'm suffering." And I also see it when people lack meaning and purpose.

Let me tell you a story about some of my colleagues. I take care of a lot of physicians, and one of the scariest things for me is to tell a surgeon, "It's not wise for you to go back and do surgery." Basically what I am saying is your career is over as you know it. This is devastating, especially in men. It is not unusual for all of us to identify who we are with what we do. And if we take away that what we do, we lose the meaning and purpose in our life. If we have no meaning and purpose, why do we get out of bed in the morning? This is crucially important. So I see people come in and tell me, "I am blue.

I am down. Why bother?" This is how it presents. Depression for example has a 40 percent higher coronary artery disease rate, and a 60 percent higher death rate.

And depression has a kissing cousin, if you might, something called hopelessness. We frequently see depression and hopelessness together. But if someone comes into the hospital and they are depressed, they do not do very well. Especially people who already have documented coronary artery disease. They are less likely to do well with surgery. They have more post-surgical complications. They have a two-fold increase risk in their outpatient mortality and a five-fold increase in death after a first heart attack. I always tell my cardiac fellows, "When you talk to our patients and they have had a heart attack, do you look at the situation of their life? Do you find out what has been going on?" Everyone is so happy to report the cholesterol level, but they forget to report if someone is depressed, if they are stressed, if they are socially isolated, if they feel hopeless, if they have given up. These are equally important and independent risk factors for disease.

Remember, we talked about this concept of the autonomic nervous system. We said that autonomic means automatic. Let's take a quick review. If our foot is on the gas all the time that means our sympathetic nervous system is revved up, we are stimulated. This is what occurs when we live under chronic stress, we have our foot on the gas. On the other side, we can have our foot on the brake that is our relaxation side to the nervous system, what we call the parasympathetic nervous system. What we really want is to have these two in balance. You can't be on the gas all the time; you can't be on the brake all the time. So they need to be in balance. And we discussed something called heart rate variability, and heart rate variability, that beat-to-beat variation between heartbeats, is an important predictor of health. As a reminder, if the heart rate variability is low, that is an independent predictor of heart attack and sudden cardiac death. If heart rate variability is high, that implies more flexibility within the autonomic nervous system, and is associated with a better outcome. And we talked about how can we modify this intentionally? We said we can modify it through our breathing, our five seconds in, five seconds out. We talked about modifying heart rate variability with Tai Chi; we talked about modifying it with prayer, and with mantra repetition. Why is it connected to depression and hopelessness? When we lose touch with who we are. The researchers believe that this is related to low heart rate variability.

It is felt that when people feel hopeless and they give up, they are less likely to comply with those things that will improve their heart rate variability, and make them healthy. You have heard me say this before, if someone is feeling hopeless, my telling them, "Go out and exercise, and eat green leafy vegetables," is probably not going to work. I need a different approach. I can't start there.

I see a lot of people who come to me after open-heart surgery. Like Ron, who I talked about, they say, "I want to get off this train track; one surgery is enough for me." But there is something else that I see, and this is not rare. People come to see me after surgery, and the best way I can describe it is they are a shell of themselves.

So what happens when someone goes through the trauma of a big surgery? It is terrifying. When I try talking to these patients, they just stare at me, and frequently the wife is next to the husband who has had the surgery, and the wife is taking notes, and the wife is telling me what medications they are on. Why? Because the person who had the surgery is just not there. In medicine, we have a kind of a nasty way of describing this; we say the lights are on, but nobody's home. But to me this is trauma; this is emotional trauma; this is shock. This is how we feel when we get bad news. One minute on my patient George. George was a big strong concrete worker, construction guy, had to have a bypass. Came back to me after his bypass and he was not the same person. We were trying everything, everything that Western medicine can give him, but he was disconnected completely. And then one day, after George had a Healing Touch treatment, I went and I whispered in his ear and I said, "George, I need you to call your spirit back." The Native Americans say, "Call your spirit back." I said, "Call it back from the operating room. Call it back from the surgeon's office. I need you to do this; I need you to want to live." And guess what happened? George came back, and he said to me, "Dr. Guarneri, of all the things you could have told me, when you told me to call my spirit back, I connected. I got what you were saying."

So how do we call our spirit back? How do I help my patients to call their spirit back? And how do you call your spirit back? It is about reconnecting with what is important in this life. It is about finding hope, establishing community, and even if we have a health challenge, change our perspective on that challenge, and ultimately we have to work toward finding inner peace.

As a holistic integrative medicine physician, I take this idea very seriously. Remember, holistic means whole. To treat the whole person, body, mind, emotions, and spirit. And just as I ask my patients, "What did you do for body, mind, emotions, and spirit today?" I address all of those issues in my practice.

We have seen a few of the tools that make integrative holistic medicine special. I could not just give my patient George a pill, I promise you, he was on every pill that was available, including antidepressants. But what makes the integrative holistic medicine approach is I have the opportunity to pick from a bigger toolbox. You have already heard about many of these tools, the first being guided imagery. Today, George would have had guided imagery tapes before he went for his bypass surgery, and he would have listened to those tapes before and after surgery, and as we showed, his chances of being in the hospital two days less were pretty high. We talked about other ways to connect body, mind, and spirit. We talked about the power of meditation. And we talked about yoga. Some of the easiest techniques we have available with us all the time. Breathing techniques, like the heart-centered breath, which we already know stops the stress response right in its tracks. Repetitive prayer and mantras, all of these techniques work to help us find inner peace.

I mentioned to you that George was receiving Healing Touch when I whispered into his ear, "Call your spirit back." Why did I send him for Healing Touch? Because I think the Healing Touch is the glue that helps to keep my patients together. That is how profound a treatment it is, and in George's case, the combination worked like magic.

And you know what? Patients want me to spend time talking about spiritual issues. Do you know an average patient appointment is 20 minutes? Yet 10 percent of patients are willing to give up time spent on their medical issues in an office visit to discuss religion and spiritual practices. Patients want to get back on track; they know it is important.

There are some other equally important aspects of spirituality that we will address. These are big ones. Forgiveness, practicing gratitude, how do I help someone get from that glass that is half empty to a glass that is half full? What we will be talking about this and one of the key steps to getting there: the power of positive thinking. Because when we put it all together, whether it is yoga and meditation, whether it is mantras and prayer, whether it is forgiveness and gratitude, we are not just healing the physical body, what we are doing is integrating everything; that is why we call it integrative medicine. We are integrating body, mind, emotions, and spirit, and even more importantly, we are saying the physical, mental, emotional aspects of healing can't be separated.

Components of Spiritual Wellness
Lecture 20

In previous lectures, you have encountered the devastating medical implications of depression, hopelessness, and even lack of social connection, but you have also learned that religion, spirituality, and social connection of all types can have a positive impact on health. In this lecture, you will be introduced to some of the components of spirituality—including forgiveness, positive thoughts, and gratitude—and you will learn some techniques to help you live a more spirited life. Forgiveness, positive thinking, and gratitude are key ingredients to healing the body, mind, and spirit, and they make for powerful medicine.

Learning to Forgive

- Learning to forgive is essential to spiritual health. Forgiveness is the very heart of spiritual counseling because it is the basis of the recovery of the true self. Even psychotherapy encourages learning to forgive.

- Sometimes people have to learn to forgive their parents, partners, and spouses. People have lists of people that they need to forgive, and the biggest forgiveness is forgiveness of oneself. Forgiveness is truly the essence of emotional as well as spiritual healing.

- Dr. Fred Luskin conducted a study at Stanford University called the Stanford Forgiveness Project, which showed that—in addition to giving us an intense feeling of peace—forgiveness teaches us to take hurt less personally and to take responsibility for how we feel.

- When we forgive, we become a hero—not a victim—in the story of our life. Forgiveness is for you; it is not for the offender. Forgiveness is about taking back your power. Forgiveness is about your healing, not about the people who hurt you.

- Forgiveness does not involve denying or minimizing the hurt; it is not about accepting unkind behavior. It is not even about forgetting that something painful happened. Forgiveness is not about reconciling with the offender.

- Dr. Luskin's research points out that forgivers have decreased blood pressure, less muscle tension, and a slower heart rate. His research also shows that people who forgive have fewer illnesses and fewer chronic conditions. Forgivers are more optimistic, less angry, and less stressed. In the Stanford study, the ability to forgive led to people feeling healthier and happier.

- To help patients forgive, physicians have to start by appealing to their rational mind. Unrepressed anger, guilt, and grief interfere with optimal well-being. Anger increases the risk of a heart attack 230 percent.

The Power of Positive Thinking

- Our thoughts can make us well, or they can make us sick. Thoughts are physical; they are alive, and they have substance—even if you do not see them. You can hurt yourself and others with your thoughts.

- Thoughts are powerful, and they influence how you feel, so you need to think about what you are thinking about. When you have negative, hurtful, hateful thoughts, you are creating the same types of negative feelings in yourself.

- The negative thoughts of hate, anger, jealousy, and envy are all problems that are associated with stress. The solution, which seems to be simple but is not, is to think positive thoughts. Positive thoughts lead to positive deeds, which lead to positive actions. Start thinking positive, nonjudgmental thoughts and start feeling positive emotions because these positive thoughts and feelings can improve your health.

- Research shows that positive thinking increases lifespan. Positive thinkers have lower rates of depression and stress, greater resistance to the common cold, reduced risk of death from cardiovascular disease, and better coping skills during hardships and times of stress.

- One of the reasons that positive thinking is so powerful is because positive outlook enables you to cope better with stressful situations, which reduces your stress hormones and the negative impact that they have on your body.

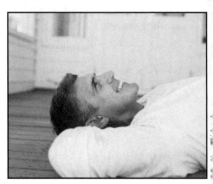

- You can start the journey of thinking positively by identifying areas that you want to change— by thinking about your thoughts. For example, if you want to become more optimistic and engage in more positive thinking, look at the

You can improve your health by thinking positive thoughts that bring about positive emotions.

situations in which you are typically negative and look at the people you interact with when you are in those negative spaces. In other words, look at who your friends are.

- Choose at least one area of your life that you are negative about, and try to approach it differently. For example, start your day by thinking about being happy to be at your job because, after all, you could always be in a worse situation. You could be heading to the hospital for surgery instead. Then, throughout the day, evaluate yourself. Stop and think about what you are thinking and what is going on in your mind. If you find that your thoughts are mainly negative, try to find a way to put a positive spin on them.

- Stop playing tapes of negative phrases and concepts over and over in your mind. You have done your best; let the past go. Do not think that you cannot do something or that you do not know how to do something because you have never done it before. Instead, look at it as an opportunity to learn something new. Find creative ways to tackle the problems and challenges in your life.

Practicing an Attitude of Gratitude
- Robert Emmons at the University of California, Davis, conducted research on gratitude and found that individuals who keep a gratitude journal on a weekly basis are healthier, exercise more, have less physical problems, and feel better overall. Grateful people report higher levels of positive emotions, greater life satisfaction, and optimism.

- Furthermore, people with a strong disposition toward gratitude have the capacity to be more empathetic and to take the perspective of others. They are also more generous.

- Keeping a gratitude journal is a great way to consciously remember and recall the things that have occurred during the day and to bring the good things to the focus, shifting your thinking to the positive. Every night, write down five things that you are grateful for in your journal. Then, write a few words about it.

- You need to practice an attitude of gratitude. It is good for your health. It changes your perception, and perception is everything.

Questions to Consider

1. Name three components of spiritual wellness.

2. Forgiveness is associated with what health benefits?

Components of Spiritual Wellness
Lecture 20—Transcript

In our previous lectures, we explored the devastating medical implications of depression, hopelessness and even the lack of social connection. But we have seen that religion and spirituality and social connection of all types can have a positive impact on our health. Today, we will explore some of the components of spirituality. Things like forgiveness, positive thoughts, and gratitude. And we will see why they make for powerful medicine.

As a holistic integrative physician, I have a different kind of training than what I got in medical school. In that training I developed a different belief system. I have truly come to believe, maybe because of my own spiritual path, that everything happens for a reason. And I believe that everything that happens to a patient can truly be an opportunity for spiritual and emotional growth. Do you know what I have patients tell me? I have them say, "Cancer is the best thing that happened to me," and I say, "Why? Why? Why could that be?" And they say, "Because when I heard those words, 'you have cancer,' everything in my life changed. I was no longer worried about the faucet that was not working 100 percent, or that the grass was an inch too high, I right away started to think about what is truly important in my life." So my goal as a physician, as a holistic physician is to promote the patient's own spirituality. I am not interested in imposing my own. I really want to meet people where they are at, and see where they want to go.

I used to call myself a plumber. Sometimes that was easier than saying I was an interventional cardiologist. And people actually reacted in a very different way. They looked at me a little unusual, "You're a plumber?" But that is really what I was. I was fixing coronary arteries with stents. I have since moved my thinking from fixing, to helping, and now most importantly to serving. This has changed my whole relationship with my patients. Actually, this concept has changed my life.

So as a physician, I ask my patients about their spiritual life and their spiritual practices. I want to know, do they have a formal meditation practice? Have they learned to take a mini moment? What is important to them? The most important question I can ask someone is what is your purpose for being here? Because I am looking for an anchor, something that makes sense about their life, to reconnect them with meaning and purpose. If they do not have a spiritual life, I may introduce the concept that spirituality is a component of optimal health, and that I would emphasize everyone's journey is unique. This is a perfect example of not one-size fits all. At the Scripps Center for Integrative Medicine, I have a little tagline that I use and it is: There are many paths to healing. Just like there are many paths to God.

What might I suggest to a patient, and where do we get started? Ultimately the goal, remember, is inner peace, how do I feel comfortable with who I am? One of the hardest things is to get people to love themselves. Do you remember when I told you the story about Ron, my patient who was 168 pounds overweight, and he lost all the weight, cured his diabetes, went from 16 medications to three medications, and I asked Ron, I said, "Ron, what was it?" and I was still naive in my thinking. I thought Ron would tell me, "Oh it was discipline, Dr. G., it was commitment, it was perseverance, it was inner strength." Do you know what he said? "I learned to love myself," he said. "I used to look in the mirror every day and see this big person that I hated. And when I finally realized that I am okay, and that I can love myself, I began to take care of my physical body."

So how do we get from there, to here? The path to inner peace may be some of the things we talked about. I know for me, it is meditation. I take my 20 minutes twice a day because meditation is medicine, and I am smiling because I had an e-mail from a patient this morning, and I had sent him to a TM meditation program, and he e-mailed me and he said, "How do you have the time for this, 20 minutes twice a day?" and I thought, oh my goodness, we have 24 hours in a day and all we are looking for is 20 minutes twice a day to give that to oneself. I think I was able to convince him.

So for me that was my path. For others, it may be just simply the breath, learning to take deep breaths to turn off the stress response. If you are one of those people that like the idea of prayer, then do your repetitive prayer. Or, if you like the concept of chanting, then go back and do it. Bring those things back into your life. There are a few other very, very powerful aspects to spiritual work. One of the biggest is forgiveness. Changing the way we think, our attitude, our mind. These are key as we begin our journey.

So let's start with one that a lot of people have difficulty with, and that is learning to forgive. Learning to forgive is essential to spiritual health. I remember once being on the big island of Hawaii, at all places a cardiology conference, a room filled with cardiologists, but the person who was hosting the conference, Dr. Earl Bakken—by the way, he is the man that invented the pace maker, a true visionary—he decided he was going to bring a kahuna, basically a spiritual teacher to this very conservative cardiology conference. So he invited a woman named Auntie Margaret, and it was amazing for me to watch, because cardiologist after cardiologist went to talk to this maybe 3'5" bit of a woman who was sitting in a wheelchair. And many of them would bend down so that they can be at her level.

So just imagine this, cardiologist after cardiologist coming to see Auntie Margaret. And she said the same thing every time, "Before the sun goes down, forgive." I do not know if it is because we were on the island of Hawaii, she said, "Go in the ocean before the sun goes down, and forgive." Her medicine was the same for everyone. Forgiveness is the very heart of spiritual counseling, because it is the basis of the recovery of the true self. Even psychotherapy is about learning to forgive. Sometimes people have to learn to forgive their parents, they have to learn to forgive their partners, their spouses. People have lists of people that they need to forgive, and the biggest forgiveness is forgiveness of oneself. Forgiveness is truly the essence of emotional as well as spiritual healing.

Dr. Fred Luskin conducted a study at Stanford University, which is called the Forgiveness Project. And basically, what he showed that forgiveness gives us, besides this intense feeling of peace, we learn to take hurt less personally. We can now take responsibility for how we feel. How many times do I hear people say to me, "So-and-so did something to me?" That makes us a victim. But when we forgive, we become a hero. We are no longer a victim in the story of our life. Now this is an important point to remember: Forgiveness is for you. It is not for the offender. Forgiveness is about taking back your power. Remember when we said we leave pieces of our spirit in traumatic places? Forgiveness is taking our power back. Forgiveness is about your healing, not about the people who hurt you.

It is equally important to recognize that forgiveness is not denying or minimizing the hurt; we are not saying it did not happen. Forgiveness is not about accepting unkind behavior. It is not about saying, "I excuse it." It is not even about forgetting that something painful has happened. Forgiveness is not reconciling with the offender. Remember, forgiveness is for you. Now Dr. Luskin's research points out that forgivers have decreased blood pressure, less muscle tension, and a slower heart rate. Well, there is no surprise to me that his research also shows people who forgive have fewer illnesses and fewer chronic conditions.

I remember a man who came into my office once, and he was totally fixated on something that happened 20 years ago. Someone did him wrong, and he was going to get them. Twenty years ago. I finally said to him, "This is like eating rat poison and expecting the rat to die." He looked at me. I said, "Who are you hurting every time you get angry?" All those emotions were coming up in anger and revenge, and I remember he kept going like this, pounding his hand on his knee, and he was going to get them. Twenty years ago this event happened. So it is no surprise to me that if I can get him to forgive, I do not expect him to forget, but if I can get him to forgive, he will have less health problems. And I know for a fact, in this case, it would cure his high blood pressure.

So what else did we learn from the Stanford study? We learned that forgivers are more optimistic; we learned that they are less angry, forgivers are less stressed, and the ability to forgive led to people feeling healthier and happier by the end of the study.

So how do I help my patients to forgive? The guy who is banging on the desk? The first thing I need to do, quite frankly, is appeal to his rational mind. It is really important to understand that unrepressed anger, guilt, and grief interfere with optimal well being. I would even show him some of the data on this. Remember, anger increases the risk of a heart attack 230 percent. I would encourage him to maybe accept some support from a counselor, from a group, even to work through his unprocessed material in a journal. People frequently say to me, "I do not know what to write, I have nothing to write." I say, "It does not matter. Get your journal, open it up, and just start writing." Or if you really feel like you can't get started, say, "What's my word for today?" and pick a word, and that word usually is about how you are feeling. To my patients that are more embedded in a spiritual path, I can more easily encourage them to surrender their pain and their suffering to a higher power.

Our mind plays a lot of tricks on us. Do you remember we talked about monkey mind? You know how monkey goes from branch to branch to branch to branch? And our mind goes from thought to thought to thought to thought? Well, we have to train our mind. Meditation is a way to train the mind.

I am going to tell you a secret: I was not always this way. I was not the person who saw the glass as half full. I had to work at it. I remember once I went to give a lecture in Wisconsin, I was at a beautiful hotel, I was being really taken care of by the nicest people, and I came out of my room, and let me describe this to you: There were trees outside, all around the hotel, and the snow was falling, and it was collecting on the branches. The first thing I thought was, "Oh no, snow storm. I will never get home; I am going to have to cancel my patients." I went right to the negative. A young woman came walking by with her boyfriend. She walked by, saw the same beautiful picture window, the same trees, the same snowfall, and she said, "Wow, isn't this beautiful?" Boy, that was a slap in the face. I needed to change my thinking. Well it is no different for my patients. Our thoughts can make us well, or our thoughts can make us sick. The native priests of Hawaii say that thoughts are physical. They are alive, and they have substance. This is true even if you do not see them. You can hurt yourself with your thoughts, and you can hurt others with your thoughts. Thoughts are powerful, and they influence how we feel, so we need to think about what we are thinking about.

One of my favorite books is Miguel Ruiz' book called *The Four Agreements*. And the first agreement is be impeccable with your word. My family used to say to me, "If you have nothing good to say, do not say it." I never realized: Do not think it. When we have negative, hurtful, hateful thoughts, we are creating the same types of negative feelings in our selves. Remember when we discussed the stress zone, the negative thoughts of hate, of anger, jealousy, envy, all of those were in that area. So the solution is simple, but it is really not so simple. It would be easy for me to say, "Think positive thoughts. Right thoughts lead to right deeds lead to right actions." Well that sounds good, but it is not really that easy. But it is what I want you to do. I want you to start thinking positive, nonjudgmental thoughts. And I also want you to start feeling those positive emotions we talked about, your newborn baby, your grandchild, your cute little puppy, all those things that bring out those positive emotions, because we have already seen in previous lectures how this can improve our health.

Thinking positive is not just this abstract concept that has not been studied. Positive thinking has been shown to increase lifespan. Positive thinkers have lower rates of depression and lower levels of stress. Positive thinkers have greater resistance to the common cold, and I have talked about a cold study. Positive thinkers have reduced risk of death from cardiovascular disease. And the research also shows that positive thinkers have better coping skills during hardships and times of stress.

So why is positive thinking so powerful? Well, the obvious one is one theory says positive outlook enables you to cope better with stressful situations. This, of course, reduces your stress hormones, and the negative impact that those have on your body. How do I do this with my patients? How do we begin to take this journey? The first thing I tell my patients to do is identify areas that they want to change. I want you to think about your thoughts. For example, if you want to become more optimistic, and engage in more positive thinking, look at those areas where you are typically negative. Are you negative about the neighbor? Are you doom and gloom about your teenagers? Is it your boss? Is it your daily commute to work? Is it your job? Where do you go to the negative? And I am going to ask you to do something else, and you know what I mean when I say this: Look at those people you interact with when you are in that negative space. We know how to find those people, because they are as negative as we are. We go and we say, "Is this not terrible?" they say, "That's terrible." "Isn't it awful?" "Oh, he is terrible." "Yep, everything's terrible." "Everything's terrible." That is it. We go and find those people when we want to get into that kind of space, we do not go and find a cheery person at the front desk who has got that overflowing glass. We go and pick people that are thinking the way we do, so the second part of this is look at who your friends are. Remember what my grandmother said: "Show me your friends, and I will show you who you are."

So pick one area, I do not expect you, if you have three areas you can't do them all at once, or maybe you can, but at least pick one. Say, "You know what? I am going to go to work and approach it differently today. I am going to go to work and I am going to be happy to be there, because, guess what? I am not going to the hospital for surgery." Right? I need you to start working on it in this way. And then throughout your whole day, evaluate yourself. Stop and think about what you are thinking, what is going on in your mind. And if you find that your thoughts are mainly negative, try to find a way to put a positive spin on them. And then I have a little trick that I like. I like to think sometimes about a golden door. I do not do it so much anymore, but I used to when I first started to shift my thinking, when I was trying to get myself out of the negative, but I used to think about a beautiful golden door with a big key in it, a golden key. And the minute my mind would go to the negative, I would imagine I put my hand on that key, and I turned the key, and as I am turning the key, I am putting a positive thought in my mind. It may just be I turn the key, and I see my niece and nephew. I turn the key, and I see my poodle. Whatever it is that makes you feel love and appreciation, you will stop the thought in a second. So I like the golden key as a way to get started.

If you are one of those people that are playing the negative tapes—oh I hate this lecture, I do not believe in spirituality, oh, what does this have to do with anything?—stop the tapes. Stop playing the negative tapes in your mind. You are good enough; you have done your best, let that past stuff go. Change the words. I teach it to my patients like this: When they say to me, "I can't do something, I do not know how to do it, I have never done it before." I say, "Do not look at it that way. Say it is an opportunity to learn something new." Wow, does not that feel better? I have an opportunity to learn something new. Another one I hear all the time, "I am not going to get any better at this." And usually when they are talking to me, they are taking about their nutrition or their lifestyle or it could be anything. And I say, "Why don't we think about it this way. Let's find a creative way to tackle this problem," or "Let's find a creative way to tackle this challenge." It feels totally different.

When we had the financial crisis hit in 2008, I watched a lot of people struggle. And my office was packed with people who had high blood pressure, who could not sleep, who were having chest pain, because they lost a lot of money. And you know what? They did not have their spiritual life in order. They still had beautiful homes, they were still healthy, they still had their spouse and their kids, but they were not counting their blessings. And when they would say to me, "I'm unemployed," I would say to them, "No, you are ready for employment." So listen to your tapes, and change the words.

We have talked about forgiveness and the power of forgiveness, and we said forgiveness is for you. It is not for the person who did something to us. And we have talked about positive thinking, but there is one other piece to the puzzle that I think is really important, which is practicing an attitude of gratitude.

Robert Emmons at UC Davis conducted some amazing research, and what he found was that individuals who keep a gratitude journal on a weekly basis are healthier, they exercise more, they have less physical problems, they feel better overall. Grateful people report higher levels of positive emotion, greater life satisfaction, and optimism. So the question is, again, is your cup half full, or half empty?

Furthermore, people with a strong disposition towards gratitude have the capacity to be more empathetic and to take the perspective of others. They are more generous. It is not just about them. This is the same as my saying, "I want you to count your blessings." A gratitude journal is a great way to go, because a gratitude journal is a way to consciously remember and recall the things that have occurred during the day and to bring the good ones to the light, so we shift our thinking to the positive.

I used to keep a gratitude journal by my bedside. I do not need to do it anymore. But take a journal, a book, and write down every night five things that you are grateful for. They can be as tiny as, "I am grateful that the sun came out." "I am grateful that I was able to walk today." That you can see; that you can hear. Write those things down. The kindness of a stranger. I am grateful for Great Courses, and all the help I have gotten to put this program together. Next, write a few words about it. I tell my patients, "If you change your thinking, you will change your life."

So, at the end of the day, we definitely need to practice an attitude of gratitude. It is good for our health. It changes our perception, and as we have decided previously, perception is everything. Together, we have looked at the power of forgiveness, positive thought, and gratitude. We have learned some techniques, the gratitude journal being one, to help us live more spirited lives.

Remember, positive thoughts, positive emotions, forgiveness, and gratitude are key ingredients to heal body, mind, and spirit.

Applying the Lessons of Natural Healing
Lecture 21

In this lecture, you are going to take what you have learned so far in this course and apply it to an actual person named Nancy. In short, you will pretend to be a holistic integrative medicine physician. You will give Nancy the powerful tools that she needs to strengthen her soil—including proper nutrition and an exercise plan. In addition, you will give her powerful stress-reduction tools and a reminder to connect with her community. Before Nancy leaves your imaginary office, make sure that she knows that you are part of her healing team.

A Case Study

- Imagine yourself as a holistic integrative medicine physician. A woman named Nancy comes in to your office to see you. She is 58 years old, and she tells you that she has a new diagnosis of diabetes, high cholesterol, and high blood pressure.

- When you ask Nancy what made her want to come in to see you, she says, "I have never been on medication before. Now, I am taking three pills: one for high blood pressure, one for diabetes, and one for high cholesterol. Is there some other way than taking all of these medications?"

- Holistic integrative medicine physicians teach to treat the whole person—body, mind, emotions, and spirit. They believe that the emotional, mental, and spiritual aspects of healing cannot be separated from the physical. They also believe that food, daily exercise, and meditation are medicine. Furthermore, they believe in the healing power of connection and touch.

- With these principles in mind, you can begin to put together all the different pieces of Nancy's story. However, before doing that, start with a physical exam.

- You find that Nancy is overweight, so you are safe to assume that her being overweight is contributing to her diabetes and high blood pressure. Her body mass index is 30, but the goal for women is less than 22.

- Nancy is wearing her weight around her midline, in the form of abdominal fat. She is shaped like an apple instead of a pear, and this shape is associated with a higher risk of heart disease. Nancy's blood pressure is 140/90, which is high because 120/80 is normal.

- Nancy's laboratory tests confirm that she does have diabetes and that her cholesterol is high. In fact, her good cholesterol, the HDL, is low, and when this is the case, the triglycerides are often high, and that is exactly what Nancy has. In addition, Nancy's LDL, the bad cholesterol, is high.

- Nancy's blood tests also show that her vitamin D level is low—so low that she is deficient. A blood test for inflammation is called an hs-CRP, and Nancy's blood test shows that she is, in fact, inflamed.

- After identifying that Nancy is overweight, has diabetes, and has signs of inflammation, you might decide to draw Nancy a picture of a tree and label three sick leaves on the branches of the tree as diabetes, high cholesterol, and high blood pressure. You might point out to Nancy that Western medicine typically goes right up to the sick leaves and either cuts them off through surgery, bypasses them through surgery, or applies pharmaceutical therapy—but that is not your approach. You might then explain to Nancy that just as the health of the tree depends on the quality of its soil, her own health depends on the soil she lives in.

- In order to strengthen Nancy's soil, you need to take a deeper look, so you should ask Nancy to tell you her story. Nancy says she is a corporate executive. She was born in Wisconsin and was raised on a farm. She describes her childhood as very happy. She was raised Catholic, and she describes herself as spiritual, but she adds that she has had no time for church because of her grueling work schedule.

- Nancy is not married and has never been married. She has no children. She tells you that she has three close friends but no pets, partner, or significant other.

- After listening to Nancy's story, you have the opportunity to ask her a few questions. You start by doing a nutrition assessment, and you discover that Nancy loves simple carbohydrates and eats a lot of sugar. She also tells you that she usually misses lunch, but she does drink at least three cups of coffee—with cream and sugar—per day. She eats less than three servings of fruits and vegetables per day and admits that her major proteins are beef and chicken.

- Nancy informs you that she has never had a food allergy, but she craves and loves dairy. By listening to Nancy, you also learn that she has gas and bloating, and sometimes it alternates with diarrhea and constipation. She describes pain in all of her joints—but especially in her hands. You have to add an additional sick leaf to Nancy's tree because she is telling you that she has arthritis.

- Nancy tells you that she drinks two glasses of red wine per night to unwind. Her aerobic exercise is less than one hour per week, and she does no strength training. In addition, Nancy has no formal stress reduction practice.

- After asking Nancy to fill out some questionnaires, you find that Nancy scored high in three areas: depression, social

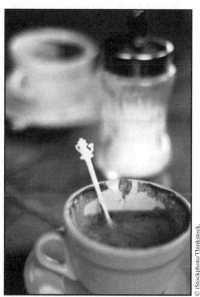

© iStockphoto/Thinkstock.

Unsweetened green tea is a great alternative to alcohol or coffee because it lowers cholesterol.

271

isolation, and perceived stress. You can now add another leaf to her tree: depression.

Putting It All Together

- The top three contributing factors to the sick leaves on Nancy's tree are her diet, lack of exercise, and stress. Start by addressing her diet; recommend a low-sugar or low-glycemic diet with no saturated fat. Specifically, you can recommend the anti-inflammatory Mediterranean diet. Eating whole foods will lower her cholesterol and blood sugar.

- If she is concerned about the amount of protein that she will get after cutting out the saturated fat that is found in the beef and chicken she frequently eats, you can recommend a protein smoothie that has soy protein, almond milk, and even omega-3 fish oil to lower her triglycerides. Also recommend adding a little bit of fiber, a handful of organic berries, and some liquid vitamin D (which will also help with depression) to her smoothie every day.

- To address Nancy's arthritis and inflammation, you should recommend that she cut back on her sugar and red meat consumption, exercise, and reduce the amount of stress she is experiencing. Because of her arthritis, gas, and bloating, Nancy probably has a sensitivity to dairy, so she should substitute cow's milk for soy milk, almond milk, or rice milk. She should also work to decrease her consumption of alcohol and caffeine by drinking water or tea instead.

- The reason that Nancy wants to be healthy is because she has to take care of her elderly parents. This is her anchor—her reason to live. Recommend repetitive prayer as a stress management tool for her. Restructure her weekend to include walking with friends and perhaps even going back to church.

1. Name three natural techniques to decrease weight and improve diabetes and high blood pressure.

2. What are some components of a mind, body, and spirit holistic integrative assessment?

Applying the Lessons of Natural Healing
Lecture 21—Transcript

Welcome back. Today is a special day. Today we are going to take what we learned so far in the science of natural healing and apply it to an actual person. In short, I want you to become a holistic integrative medicine physician.

Imagine yourself in the office and a woman comes in to see you. Her name is Nancy. Nancy is 58-years-old, and she tells you she has a new diagnosis of diabetes, high cholesterol, and high blood pressure. When you ask Nancy what made her want to come and see you, she says, "I have never been on medication before. Now I am on three pills, one for high blood pressure, one for diabetes, and one for high cholesterol. Is there some other way than taking all of these medicines?"

We are really happy Nancy asked that question, and we are equally happy that she came in to see us, aren't we? Because in our paradigm of health we no longer just talk about diseases, that is the old way, the ill to the pill. Nancy was diagnosed with three ills, so she has been given three pills. This is holistic integrative medicine and this is the science of natural healing, so we definitely have another way.

Let's review some of the basic principles of holistic integrative medicine. Remember we teach to treat the whole person, body, mind, emotions, and spirit. We believe the emotional, mental, and spiritual aspects of healing can't be separated from the physical. We believe food, daily activity, and meditation is medicine. And, we believe in the healing power of connection and touch.

With these principles in mind we begin to put together all the different pieces of Nancy's story. But, before we do that, let's take a step back, let's go back to some basics and do a physical exam.

We find that Nancy is overweight, and we are already thinking, is her being overweight contributing to her diabetes? Her high blood pressure? We know it is. Her body mass index is 30, and remember the goal for women is less than 22. We also notice something else about Nancy: She is wearing her weight around her midline, in the form of abdominal fat. We make a note that Nancy is shaped like an apple instead of a pear. We also know that this shape is associated with a higher risk of heart disease. We checked Nancy's blood pressure and find it is indeed high, 140/90, and remember we said 120/80 is normal.

Nancy's laboratory tests give us lots of information. They confirm that she does have diabetes. They also confirm that her cholesterol is high. In fact, her good cholesterol, the HDL, is low. And you remember that when the HDL is low, the triglycerides frequently go high, and that is exactly what Nancy has. In addition, Nancy's LDL—remember we said lousy cholesterol—is also high. We notice two other things in Nancy's blood tests, the first is that her vitamin D level is low, so she has vitamin D deficiency, and this is really important. We also notice something else, there is a special blood test for inflammation, and that blood test is called an HS CRP. That blood test is high, so that tells us that Nancy is inflamed.

So now we are thinking Nancy is overweight, she has diabetes, and she already has signs of inflammation. So we decide to draw Nancy a picture of a tree, and we go up to the branches and we label three sick leaves on the tree. We call them diabetes, high cholesterol, and high blood pressure. We point out to Nancy that Western medicine typically goes right up to the sick leaves and either cuts them off through surgery, bypasses them through surgery, or applies pharmaceutical therapy. We explain to Nancy that that is not our approach. We explain to her that just as the health of the tree depends on the quality of its soil, her own health depends on the soil she lives in. What is the quality of her soil?

So up until now, we really have the truncated or shortened version of Nancy's story, do we not? We know a few things: We have problems that have been labeled, diabetes, high blood pressure, and high cholesterol. But those are just names. So we made a diagnosis, but in order to strengthen Nancy's soil, we need to take a deeper look, do we not? So we asked Nancy to tell us her story.

Nancy begins to tell us her story, and she starts with her work. She says she is a corporate executive. She was born in Wisconsin and raised on a farm. She describes her childhood as very happy. She had no medical problems as a child. Her mom stayed at home and raised Nancy and her two siblings. She describes the household as happy. She was raised Catholic, and she describes herself as spiritual, but she adds she has had no time for church, and has no time for spiritual practice. So we are thinking here about adverse childhood events, and we are not hearing any. Nancy, it sounds like, had a really happy childhood, but it seems like maybe she got a little disconnected from her spiritual practices because of her work.

What else do we learn from Nancy? Nancy tells us she left home to attend university at the age of 17. She completed a Masters in Business Administration, and she is the CEO of a start-up company. She describes her workdays as long, and she eats out in restaurants most nights. Nancy tells us she is not married and has never been married. She has no children. We ask about her friends, and she tells us that she has three close friends, and that is her main social network. She has no pets at home, and no partner or significant other, and she adds, "Who has the time?"

As we listen to Nancy's story, we are listening for clues, something that will give us some insight that can be used to turn the course of her health challenges around. So we now have the opportunity to ask Nancy a few questions.

Since we have been saying all along in the science of natural healing that food comes first we want to know, what is Nancy eating? So we do a nutrition assessment, and we find that Nancy loves simple carbohydrates, and she eats lots of sugar. This includes granola, bagels at the office, and muffins at the office. Nancy tells us, "I eat whatever the staff brings in." Nancy also tells us that she usually misses lunch, and again says, "I'm too busy." But she does drink coffee, at least three cups a day, and she puts in sugar and cream. She eats less than three servings of fruits and vegetables a day, and says her major protein is almost always beef and chicken.

Nancy informs us that she has never had a food allergy, and she has never heard the term food sensitivity. So we ask Nancy, "Do you crave any foods?

Is there a food that you really like?" And she right away says, "Dairy. I love things like cheese, cottage cheese." Remember she says, "I come from Wisconsin." By listening to Nancy we also learn that she has a couple of other important symptoms. Let's go through those. She tells us she has gas and bloating, and sometimes it alternates with diarrhea and constipation. She describes pain in her joints, all her joints, but especially her hands. Well we are now thinking we have to add an additional sick leaf to Nancy's tree, because Nancy is telling us she has arthritis, so that gives us four medical challenges to address: Diabetes, high blood pressure, high cholesterol, and now arthritis.

We ask Nancy some more questions because we want to know more about her lifestyle. Fortunately, she tells us she has never smoked a cigarette, and that is really great because cigarette smoking is one of the biggest risk factors for a woman to have a heart attack.

Nancy tells us she drinks two glasses of red wine per night, and she adds, "It helps me to unwind." Her aerobic exercise is less than one hour per week, and she does no strength training. Nancy has no formal stress reduction practice. When we ask about this, she reminds us of her very busy schedule.

Let's stop for a moment and think about what we are hearing. What do you think about those two glasses of wine per night? Remember wine is pure sugar, but even more concerning, Nancy is using the alcohol to help manage her stress. Remember what she said, "It helps me to unwind." And we know for women, two drinks of alcohol a night is two too many. The maximum should be maybe three to four drinks per week, and she is well above that.

What about Nancy's lack of exercise? Well that is adding to every single sick leaf that she has on her tree. Everything she has, diabetes, high blood pressure, high cholesterol, everything would get better with exercise.

So now we know a little bit about Nancy's physical body, we know some of her habits, her nutrition, her exercise, and her use of alcohol. We now ask Nancy if she would be willing to fill out some questionnaires to help us better assess her emotional, mental, and even spiritual status, and she readily agrees. I bet you can guess the results. Nancy scored high in three areas. She scored high in depression, high in social isolation, and high in perceived stress, so we now have one more leaf to add to our tree, and that is called depression.

We now have a lot of important information about Nancy. So let's start to think about how do we put this all together as integrative holistic medicine physicians and make some truly life-saving recommendations. And yet let's use all of the knowledge that we learned in the science of natural healing. Remember we are going to care for Nancy as a whole person, body, mind, emotions, and spirit. So let's get started.

Let's look at what is contributing to those sick leaves on Nancy's tree, and let's pick the top three that will influence every one of those sick leaves: Her diet, her lack of exercise, and stress.

What do we recommend? Let's go back to the beginning—food first. Let's identify Nancy's problems. She has diabetes, her triglycerides, remember, are high, and that is the form of fat that comes from sugar. Her LDL, the bad cholesterol, is also high, and that is the form of fat that comes from saturated fat, so we recommend a low-sugar or low-glycemic diet, but we also want to eliminate the saturated fat. Isn't this sounding like the anti-inflammatory Mediterranean diet? Let's take a look at it. So we tell Nancy, "We want you to eat foods that are low in sugar. We want you to pick fruits and vegetables that are low on the glycemic index, things like apples, peaches, pears, and plums. And we definitely do not want you to eat anything white, except for maybe cabbage and cauliflower. And they are not truly, truly white. But certainly no refined sugar and no simple carbohydrates." Fortunately, Nancy tells us she likes beans and lentils. So we encourage her to eat them, and to eat them as a good source of protein, because these whole foods we have learned, and we know are going to lower her cholesterol, and lower her blood sugar. And we do have to remind Nancy about saturated fat, remember Nancy told us her main fat is chicken and beef, so we tell her that beef, pork, and lamb, cream and full-fat dairy is not a good thing for her health, and she understands.

Nancy looks a little bit concerned, and she tells us that she is worried she may not get enough protein if she is going to limit her carbohydrates. So we reinforce that we want her to eat complex carbohydrates, healthy carbohydrates, like green leafy vegetables, but because of her concerns, we recommend a protein smoothie, and then we come up with a really creative idea. Can we make a smoothie that can lower Nancy's triglycerides and her cholesterol? You bet we can. So we recommend a smoothie that has soy protein, almond milk, we tell Nancy she can put her omega-3 fish oil in the smoothie. Remember, we said four grams of omega-3 will lower triglycerides 50 percent. We also recommend a little bit of fiber, and a handful of her favorite berries, and we want her to buy them organic. We tell her she can have the berries frozen so they are like ice cubes if she enjoys her smoothie cold. Now, we know from Nancy's blood test that her vitamin D level is low, so we add some liquid vitamin D, and we give her a few drops in her smoothie every day. We have just created a smoothie that will lower triglycerides, lower cholesterol, give Nancy a nice protein boost, and not put weight on her. And we remind her, "Go slow with the fiber, because fiber can sometimes make gas and bloating worse." We recommend only three grams at this time, but we know our goal is 35 grams a day. And with the whole foods we are going to work our way to that goal.

There is one other piece to Nancy's story that sparked our attention, and I bet you are thinking about it. We put a leaf up on the tree that said arthritis, and that told us that Nancy had inflammation. She told us she had inflammation because she said her joints were hurting. The blood test confirmed the inflammation; that was the blood test called the HS CRP, and that was high. So let's review some of the potential causes of inflammation in Nancy. Remember we said midline weight produces inflammatory cytokines; so just having your weight in the midline can make you inflamed. We talked about lots of food causes of inflammation, and we said number one was sugar, and Nancy is consuming lots of sugar. Nancy is also not exercising, she is eating red meat (which is pro-inflammatory), and even stress can lead to inflammation. But there is one other thing going on, that combination of arthritis that Nancy has and that gas and bloating, and we suspect that Nancy has a sensitivity to dairy. So because of the gas and bloating, and the arthritis, we tell Nancy that we suspect she has a dairy sensitivity. She also gave us another clue to this: She told us the one food she craves all the time is—what?—dairy. And remember this pearl, the food we probably should avoid is the one we crave the most. That is one of the principles of food sensitivity. So we also ask Nancy to avoid cow's milk, cow's cheese, and substitute soymilk or almond milk or rice milk. She can even have small amounts of soy cheese, but a little bit, because some of them can have a high calorie content.

I also ask Nancy to decrease her alcohol and her caffeine. Remember the alcohol is sugar, and the caffeine in some people can really increase blood pressure, so basically what we are doing with Nancy, and we are not even calling it this, is she is going to have a real detox. She is going to decrease the alcohol, decrease the caffeine, clear out the cow's milk, clear out the sugar; this is going to be a major, major but wonderful change.

Now we know something that is a little bit of a trick, and we tell Nancy, "Decrease the alcohol and caffeine by 50 percent," because we know if we say just stop it, we may not have success. We give Nancy one other food tip: We want her to stay very hydrated—plenty of water throughout the day. And if she likes tea, we recommend green tea, because remember, green tea lowers cholesterol. But we tell her unsweetened green tea. We encourage her to avoid eating anything in a can or a package. Why? Because most of these processed foods are really high in sodium. So if she decides to eat something that is not a whole food, she needs to look at that label, and look at the sodium content, and keep that sodium below 1500 milligrams per day, because we know that the low sodium diet can really reduce high blood pressure.

What else can we do? What else can we offer Nancy at this point? We certainly need to talk about exercise, because every issue that Nancy has will be improved with exercise. We explain to Nancy that exercise lowers blood pressure and helps us to decrease our weight. We also explain that she might not be fully ready for a big exercise program because she has not done exercise in a long time. So we start easy and we give her a pedometer, and we tell her that her goal is 10,000 steps a day. How does she get there? Well we make some easy recommendations. Park the car further away, take the steps and not the elevator, and make time in the mid-day to walk for at least a half an hour. We also know that the exercise is going to lower Nancy's blood sugar, and exercise is a treatment for depression.

But we don't stop there; those are just the physical body recommendations. Remember, we are holistic integrative medicine physicians and we have identified that Nancy has some concerns, one is social isolation, another is stress, and the third being depression. We recognize that her vitamin D level was low, and we know that low vitamin D is linked to depression. So we added the vitamin D into her smoothie, and we have seen that Nancy has a religious and spiritual belief system, but it really has not been integrated into her life.

So let's think about stress. Nancy is quick to tell us that she is concerned about taking time out of her day for stress reduction. I do not have time for stress reduction, she says. We remind her that stress is one of the key ingredients, like lack of exercise, causing all of her problems. She looks a little bit surprised. We tell her that stress leads to weight in the midline. We tell her that stress leads to mindless eating. We just eat and we do not pay attention sometimes to what we are even doing. We also tell her that stress raises cholesterol and raises her blood pressure. Nancy now looks at us because she is beginning to understand what has been going on. And as she begins to soften, we ask Nancy a really important question. We ask her, "What is the most important thing in your life? What makes you want to get better? What makes you want to live?" Because after all, she came in to see us for a reason. At this point Nancy actually begins to cry. She tells us that she really wants to stay well to take care of her elderly parents, and she says, "They were so good to me growing up, I had every opportunity in life." So we have found Nancy's anchor, her reason to live. We recommend repetitive prayer as a stress management tool for her. She was raised Catholic, and she tells us, "This feels right." We restructure her weekend to include walking with friends and maybe even going back to church.

As Nancy gets ready to leave, we review her program. We have given Nancy powerful tools to strengthen her soil. Proper nutrition, micronutrients like vitamin D, a powerful smoothie, she knows to give up sugar and sodium. We gave her a pedometer, which she now has on her waist, and a walking plan. We did not stop there; in addition we gave her powerful stress reduction tools, and a reminder to connect with community. Before Nancy leaves our office, we give her our secret ingredient, and it is love, and it is in the form of a big hug, and we let her know we are part of her healing team.

Ecology and Health
Lecture 22

E cology is the study of all interconnected systems on the planet. In its broadest definition, what is personal is universal. In this lecture, you will learn about the findings of the Millennium Ecosystem Assessment and how climate change, the industrialization of food, and the liberal use of synthetic chemicals and plastics are altering the health of humans and the health of our planet. You will also get some glimpses into some of the steps that we can take to start improving both our health and our planet's health.

The Millennium Ecosystem Assessment

- The Millennium Ecosystem Assessment was called for by United Nations Secretary-General Kofi Annan in 2000. Over 2,000 authors and reviewers worldwide contributed their knowledge, time, and insight to this document. The objective was to assess the consequences of ecosystem change for human well-being and then to establish the scientific basis for action needed to enhance the conservation and sustainable use of ecosystems and their contributions to human well-being.

- The Millennium Ecosystem Assessment Report cited the following.
  o Twenty-five percent of mammals and 30 percent of amphibians are threatened with extinction.

  o Two-thirds of major marine fisheries are fully exploited, overexploited, or even depleted.

  o Ninety percent of the total weight of the ocean's largest predators has disappeared.

  o One billion people lack access to fresh, clean water.

- The report concluded that human activity is putting a colossal strain on the Earth's ecosystems. As humans, we can no longer ignore the fact that our health is intimately linked to the health of the planet.

Planetary Changes and Human Health
- The intragovernmental panel on climate change published a report in 2007. In the United States, the panel predicts that Chicago will experience 25 percent more frequent heat waves and that Los Angeles will experience a four- to eight-fold increase in heat wave days by the end of the century. Heat stress is bad for humans and can lead to large death tolls.

- Climate change is not just about heat. The panel also stated that the movement of homes to areas where we have to rely on automobiles and the use of the agricultural industry of land has resulted in air quality disruption.

- Between 1960 and 1990, the number of people working outside of their counties increased by over 200 percent. Although it seems like a good intention to move out of cities to be surrounded by more green land and trees, this has resulted in vehicle miles traveled increasing by 250 percent from 1960 to 1997.

- The average American driver spends 443 hours each year behind the wheel of a car, which is equivalent to about 11 weeks of work. Urban outdoor air pollution is estimated to cause 1.3 million deaths worldwide per year, and those individuals living in middle-income countries are disproportionately experiencing this burden.

- Air pollution is one of the largest contributors to cardiovascular disease. Studies of mice show that even animals on a high-fat diet do alright in terms of plaque formation, but they get sick and form more plaque—nearly double the amount—if they are given a high-fat diet combined with air pollution.

- In 1996, the Atlanta Olympic Games were taking place in the downtown area, and a decision was made to limit automobile use in the area. Automobile use was reduced by 22.5 percent, and subsequently, hospital admissions for asthma in the area decreased by 41 percent.

- Another contributor to poor air quality is the agricultural industry. In 2006, The Food and Agriculture Organization of the United Nations stated that livestock production contributed 18 percent of world greenhouse gas emissions—which is more than transportation. More recent research suggests that the livestock contribution may be as high as 51 percent of all greenhouse emissions.

- Another interesting study in 2006 at the University of Chicago concluded that a person switching from a typical American diet to a vegan diet—a diet without animal meat, eggs, or even milk— with the same number of calories would prevent the emission of 1,485 kilograms of carbon dioxide. The difference obtained by that change exceeds that of an individual switching from a Toyota Camry to a hybrid Toyota Prius.

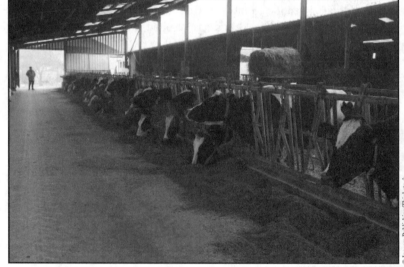

If many people switched to a vegan diet—one without animal meat, eggs, or milk—it would have a profound impact on greenhouse gas emissions.

- The livestock industry may also be affecting human health in another way. Very frequently, animals are kept on feedlots, which are confined quarters, instead of being able to graze freely in the grass. Because of this, they are routinely given antibiotics to prevent infection—not to treat sick animals. This is a true misuse of antibiotics.

- Antibiotics are a true medical miracle and are to be used when needed in the correct way. People should take antibiotics when they need them, but the use of antibiotics is becoming increasingly liberal.

- The agricultural industry uses approximately 71 percent of the antibiotics produced in the United States, and there is a strong link between antibiotics used in agriculture and antibiotic-resistant bacteria.

- A report from 2000 looked at an antibiotic-resistant salmonella outbreak that occurred in the United Kingdom. It traced the outbreak to a dairy farm where a particular antibiotic was used the month before the outbreak. The use of the antibiotic in the dairy resulted in resistant infections in humans.

- The American Society for Microbiology, the American Public Health Association, and the American Medical Association have called for substantial restrictions on antibiotic use in animal food production. They are calling for an end to all nontherapeutic uses of antibiotics in livestock.

- The other problem is that animals are being fed corn and other grains that are high in omega-6. These grains raise the omega-6 to omega-3 ratio. Because of this, meat—primarily red meat—is recognized as being proinflammatory.

Environmental Toxins
- In 2009, the Centers for Disease Control and Prevention (CDC) published the fourth national report on human exposure to

environmental chemicals. The CDC measured 212 chemicals in people's blood or urine, 75 of which have never been measured in the U.S. population before. These new chemicals include arsenic, environmental phenols, and bisphenol A.

- Bisphenol A (BPA) is an industrial chemical that has been used to make plastics and resins since the 1960s. These plastics are often used in containers that store our food and beverages, such as canned foods and baby formula cans. The health concern is that the BPA that lines cans and bottles can seep into our food.

- The American Chemistry Council is an association that represents plastic manufacturers, and they say that BPA poses no threat to human health. However, the U.S. Department of Health and Human Services and the Food and Drug Administration say that they have some concerns about the possible health effects of BPA.

- The Environmental Working Group is raising consumers' level of consciousness about this issue, and they are placing educational information in the hands of consumers to help them make clearer decisions.

Questions to Consider

1. Name two ways in which human health is linked to the planet's health.

2. How is the agriculture industry affecting human health?

Ecology and Health
Lecture 22—Transcript

Ecology is more than environmental science. Ecology is the study of all interconnected systems on the planet. In the broadest definition, what is personal is universal. Today, we will discuss the Millennium Assessment Findings, and how climate change, the industrialization of food, and the liberal use of synthetic chemicals and plastics are altering the health of humans and the health of our planet.

Let's start by looking at the Millennium Assessment Report. The Millennium Ecosystem Assessment was called for by United Nations Secretary-General Kofi Annan in 2000. Over 2000 authors and reviewers worldwide contributed their knowledge, time, and insight to this document. The objective of the Millennium Assessment was to assess the consequences of ecosystem change for human wellbeing, and then to establish the scientific basis for action needed to enhance the conservation and sustainable use of ecosystems and their contributions to human wellbeing.

In the Millennium Assessment Report, they cited the following: 25 percent of mammals and 30 percent of amphibians are threatened with extinction. Two-thirds of major marine fisheries are fully exploited, over-exploited, or even depleted. Ninety percent of the total weight of the ocean's largest predators has disappeared. And one billion people lack access to fresh, clean water.

The Millennium Assessment bottom line, and I quote, "At the heart of this assessment is a stark warning: Human activity is putting such strain on the natural functions of Earth that the ability of the planet's ecosystems to sustain future generations can no longer be taken for granted."

Well, all of that sounds pretty scary to me, and I almost want to not have to think about it. But, as a physician, and as a human on the planet, I can no longer ignore the fact that human health is intimately linked to the health of the planet. Let's take a look at some planetary changes that we are seeing right now that are linked to human health and wellbeing.

The intra-governmental panel on climate change published a report in 2007. This report stated

Climate change may directly affect human health through increases in average temperature. Rising average temperatures were predicted to increase the incidence of heat waves and heat extremes. This change in weather will affect humans both directly, the consequences of heat and indirectly, through changes in water, changes in air, and food quality.

In the United States the panel predicts that Chicago will experience 25 percent more frequent heat waves, and Los Angeles a four- to eight-fold increase in heat wave days by the end of the century. Heat stress is bad for humans, and we have important instances already that show this. During the summer of 1995 we had the Chicago Heat Wave, which claimed the lives of over 600 people. But even more remarkably in August of 2003, 45,000 people died of heat stress in Western Europe.

But climate change is not just about heat. The panel also stated,

> Climate change is expected to contribute to some air quality problems as well. Respiratory disorders may be exacerbated, as there is an increase in smog events, higher temperatures lead to worse air quality. The warming up of the climate and worsening of air quality is even further exacerbated by urbanization.

The movement of homes to areas where we have to rely on automobiles and the use of the agricultural industry of land has resulted in air quality disruption.

Between 1960 and 1990 the number of people working outside their counties increased over 200 percent. This is one of my areas that I think about as good intentions but dangerous consequences. We think it is good to move out of the cities to get more of nature and green land and trees, but this has resulted in vehicle miles traveled increasing 250 percent from 1960 to 1997. The average American driver spends 443 hours each year behind the wheel of a car. That is equivalent to around 11 weeks of work.

Urban outdoor air pollution is estimated to cause 1.3 million deaths worldwide per year, and those individuals living in middle-income countries are disproportionately experiencing this burden.

And air pollution is one of the largest contributors to cardiovascular disease. Studies done in mice show us that even animals on a very high fat diet do okay in terms of plaque formation, but they get sick and form more plaque—almost the amount—if they get the high fat diet and air pollution combined. Nearly double the amount of plaque as those that inhale filtered air. So why, as a cardiologist, do we not add to our list "air pollution" as a cause of coronary artery disease?

An interesting experiment was done for the Atlanta Olympic Games in 1996. The Atlanta Olympic Games were happening in downtown and a decision was made to limit automobile use in the area. Automobile use was reduced by 22.5 percent, but what was so insightful is that someone was measuring hospital admissions for asthma. And what they found was asthma admissions to the Atlanta ER decreased 41 percent. We know that asthma and heart disease are clearly linked to poor quality of air.

Another contributor to poor air quality as we mentioned is the agricultural industry. The way we farm is having a serious impact on the environment. The UN Food and Agricultural Organization in 2006 stated that livestock production contributed 18 percent of world greenhouse gas emissions. This is more than transportation. More recent research suggests that the livestock contribution may be as high as 51 percent of all greenhouse emissions.

Another interesting study in 2006 at the University of Chicago concluded that a person switching from a typical American diet to a vegan diet—that is a diet without animal meat, eggs, or even milk—switching from a typical American diet to a vegan diet with the same number of calories would prevent the emission of 1485 kg of carbon dioxide. The difference obtained by that, that change in diet, exceeds that of an individual switching from a Toyota Camry to the hybrid Toyota Prius. If many of us would just take this step it would have a profound impact on greenhouse gas emissions.

The livestock industry may also be affecting human health in another way. Very frequently, animals are kept on what are called feedlots. Animals are not grazing in the grass, they are kept in confined quarters, and because they are kept in confined quarters, they are routinely given antibiotics to prevent infection. Now I want to say that again: The antibiotics they get are to prevent infection. It would be like piling a lot of people in a room and we would all be breathing on each other, and we would take antibiotics to protect each other from getting sick. This is not to treat a sick animal; this is a true misuse of antibiotics. But what is really shocking here is that the agricultural industry uses approximately 71 percent of the antibiotics produced in the United States. This is important because there is a strong link between antibiotics used in agriculture and antibiotic resistant bacteria. This link has already been established. A report from 2000 looked at an antibiotic resistant salmonella outbreak that occurred in the UK. It traced the outbreak to a dairy farm where a particular antibiotic was used the month before the outbreak. The use of the antibiotic in the dairy resulted in resistant infections in humans. A similar study in 1987 reportedly traced tetracycline-resistant salmonella back to the top dressing of cattle feed. So these antibiotics are put on top of the food, they are added to the water, and in both of these cases they resulted in an antibiotic-resistant salmonella. Now, antibiotics are a true medical miracle, to be used when needed in the right way. We all know this. We tell our patients: Take your full course of antibiotics. We do not give antibiotics, for example, for viral infections. We want them when we need them, and what we are starting to see is this liberal use, 71 percent of all the antibiotics made for the U.S. are going to the agricultural industry.

There has been a call to restrict antibiotic use in animal agriculture in the United States. The American Society for Microbiology, the American Public Health Association, and the American Medical Association have called for substantial restrictions on antibiotic use in animal food production. They are calling for an end to all non-therapeutic use of antibiotics in livestock. And, more recently, a letter signed by medical professional organizations and sent to Congress in 2011 stated, and I quote,

The evidence is so strong of a link between misuse of antibiotics and food, or in animal food, and human antibiotic resistance that FDA and Congress should be acting much more boldly and urgently to protect those vital drugs for human illness.

But, we have another problem. The other problem is this, so we have animals on feedlots, they are not grazing in the grass, they are together, they are being fed antibiotics, and what they are also being fed is corn, and other grains which are high in omega-6. These grains raise the omega-6 to omega-3 ratio, and we have talked a lot about the importance of this ratio and how meat is now recognized, particularly red meat, as being pro-inflammatory.

So our food is being greatly impacted; it is affecting us, and the food industry is affecting the planet. But there is one last topic that I feel compelled to discuss, and that is the topic of environmental toxins. This is a very large area, and I invite you if this is an area of interest, go to the Environmental Working Group website, remember we talked about this, when we talked about how do we know which foods we absolutely have to buy organic and which foods we can maybe not buy organic, well that website will give lots of information: what cosmetics to purchase, which toothpaste to use, and the list goes on and on.

So, let's take a look at what the CDC found. In 2009, the Center for Disease Control published the fourth national report on human exposure to environmental chemicals. The CDC measured 212 chemicals in people's blood or urine. What was really scary to me as a physician about this report is 75 of these chemicals have never been measured in the U.S. population before. These new chemicals include things like arsenic, environmental phenols, and bisphenol A. Now, there is a large list of toxins; the CDC found 212. And what we frequently hear is something is okay, we tested it, but what routinely isn't done is things aren't tested in combination. What happens when we get exposed to three or four of these toxins? No one is looking at that, and that really concerns me, because if we do not look at the synergistic effects, even small doses begin to add up. So what might not seem like a lot could be a big problem.

Let's take a look at one of those chemicals that the CDC found, and that is called bisphenol A, also known as BPA. Now, this is an industrial chemical that has been used to make plastics and resins since the 1960s. Where do we find these chemicals? Well, these plastics are often used in containers that store our food: containers that store our beverages such as water bottles, baby bottles, and cups. Baby toys are even made out of this chemical. We find epoxy resins coating the inside of metal cans. When you open your can and you see that shine, this is the resin. So canned foods, baby formula cans, all contain BPA. The health concern is that the BPA that is lining the cans, that is lining the water bottles, can seep into our food, and this has become a very big concern for all of the holistic physicians that I know.

Now, the American Chemistry Council is an association that represents plastic manufacturers, and they say that BPA poses no threat to human health; we do not have to worry about it. But I invite you to look a little further into this, because the Department of Health and Human Services says it has some concern about the possible health effects of BPA, and they are not alone, the Food and Drug Administration agrees with them. I always like to look at what is going on in Canada. I just have the feeling that the Canadians are a little bit ahead of us in this game. They are a little bit quicker to respond to these concerns, and Health Canada's Food Directorate has concluded that the current dietary exposure to BPA through food packaging uses is not expected to pose a health risk to the general population, however—and this is a big however—they go on to make their final recommendation, and they say: Why don't limit BPA use, especially in things that our children are exposed to until there is further research?

So the toxin story is not over. And there are many more toxins that we can look at. Naphthalates, for example, in cosmetics, the list goes on and on, and fortunately we have groups in this country that are not just taking "no problem" as an answer. And, as I talked about briefly, the Environmental Working Group is one of those groups, and they are actually raising consumers' level of consciousness about this issue, and they are placing tools in the hands of the educated consumer with good backing information that helps us to make clearer decisions. I can't help but feeling, in our country, that our children are the canary in the coalmine. The most vulnerable people are the elderly and the young. And I do not know about you, but I do not feel right about having BPA in my plastic water bottle. As a matter of fact, I do not want to have it in any bottle, and certainly not in a bottle that we are going to give our children.

All of this leads up to some pretty scary stuff. We talked about just one toxin, we talked about climate change, we talked about how temperatures are warming up, and this is actually increasing deaths related to heat stress. We talked about how climate change, the rising of temperature, is affecting our air quality, and with that, we see an increase of things like heart disease and asthma.

But we got some glimpses today into some things that we can do. Remember Atlanta? They got people to stop driving cars. I went to the Beijing Olympics and I was there for a week, and they had no cars coming into the city, they really cut the automobiles down. They did that intentionally, to try to clean the air. But the week that I was there, I never got to see the sky, because of the cloud of smog. But there are good things that we can do, and there are things that we can do right now. I do not want you to leave this lecture and feel hopeless or depressed or just say, "Forget about it." I want you to think about the next seven generations, our children, and our grandchildren, and the world to come. Because we know that if we take the things we know now—maybe you are going to become a vegan, that would be a great thing—we can immediately start to improve the health of the planet.

So let's remember where we started, we said ecology is the interconnectedness of everything. It is a big matrix, stuff just does not disappear; plastic just does not go away. What is personal is universal, our health is intimately related to the health of the planet, and it is a delicate dance that we have to take together.

Healthy People, Healthy Planet
Lecture 23

In the previous lecture, you learned about some of the key factors that affect the health of humans and the health of the planet. This lecture will teach you how to take action. As an individual, you can choose to become vegan instead of eating dairy and red meat. You can also choose to filter your water instead of buying plastic water bottles. There are also changes that are happening at a larger level—both institutionally and nationally. When you make the right choices for your own health, you are also making choices that are right for planet Earth.

Acting Locally

- There are many steps that you can take immediately that will impact not only your own health, but also the health of the planet.

- One of the first things that you can do is buy organic fruits and vegetables whenever possible. Over 450 pesticides and herbicides are used on nonorganic products. Nonorganic products may be irradiated, and they have nitrates. Furthermore, the seeds of nonorganic products may even be genetically modified.

- Farmers that keep using soil over and over again deplete it of its nutrients. However, organic farmers practice crop rotation, which gives the soil more time to replenish its nutrients after producing crops. An added advantage of buying organic produce is to support organic farmers.

- A 2006 study revealed detectible metabolites of organophosphate pesticide residues in children eating a conventional diet. When these children were taken off of their conventional diet and placed on an organic diet, there were no detectible metabolites.

- In addition to buying organic whenever possible, do your best to avoid eating meat and dairy. These foods are high in saturated fat, which contributes to heart disease and inflammation. In addition, the industrialized reduction of livestock leads to increased greenhouse gas admissions.

- When you go to the supermarket, look for eggs that are free range and omega-3. If you choose to eat poultry, look for poultry that is free range and free of antibiotics and hormones—especially if you have small children. Ideally, buy organic eggs and poultry.

- If you choose to eat fish, make sure it is wild caught, such as wild sockeye salmon or wild trout. The more fat that is on the fish, the more toxins that are in the fat.

- In a study that was published in *Science* in 2004, researchers found that farm-raised Atlantic salmon had significantly higher levels of 13 toxins when compared with wild Pacific salmon. The study also measured toxin levels in the salmon chow, a mixture of ground-up fish and oil that was fed to the farm-raised salmon. They found a strong correlation between the toxicities of the chow and the salmon and concluded that the toxins were being passed into the salmon from their food.

- Fish farms use chemicals as disinfectants to kill bacteria. They use herbicides to prevent the overgrowth of vegetation in ponds, vaccines to fight certain diseases, and drugs—usually combined in the feed—to treat diseases and parasites.

Personal Changes
- Policy change plays a large role in changing the planet for the better, but individuals can also effect change very quickly. You can start by becoming vegan because vegan food is the best food that you can eat for the planet.

- Start figuring out which plastic bottles that you use contain BPA. If your bottle has a label, look underneath the bottle, and if you see the recycle number seven, it contains BPA.

- In addition, most aluminum cans are lined with BPA, so whenever possible, filter your water and select stainless-steel canisters.

- Don't put hot foods in plastic because if you do, the toxins from the plastic will seep into your food. Instead, use glass or porcelain. For the same reason, do not microwave plastic.

- One of the biggest sources of plastic is in the environment. Plastic constitutes 90 percent of all trash floating in the world's oceans. In some areas of the ocean, the amount of plastic outweighs the amount of plankton by a ratio of six to one. The truth is that, despite recycling, many of the plastic bottles that you use end up in the water.

- The Pacific garbage patch is a trash vortex that spins around; it is a gyre of ocean litter that is located in the North Pacific Ocean. The exact size of the vortex is unknown, but estimates range from an area the size of the state of Texas to one larger than the continental United States.

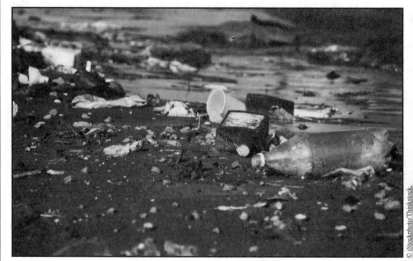

Plastic is bad for the environment and for your health, and even if you recycle plastic, you could be contributing to pollution.

- Not only is plastic bad for our health and for the planet, but plastic is also bad for animals. The albatross are dying because they are eating the plastic that human beings discard, including plastic bottle caps.

- Each year, it takes 17 billion barrels of oil and produces 2.5 billion tons of carbon dioxide pollution to produce the 30 billion plastic bottles Americans use. It also takes three times the amount of water to produce a bottle as it does to fill it. Additionally, there is a high cost associated with the transportation of those heavy bottles.

- Another simple thing that you can do to help yourself and the planet is to walk or bike instead of drive. Walking is medicine; it can improve your weight, cholesterol, depression, and even sleep.

Institutional and National Changes

- In 1998, Denmark eliminated nontherapeutic antibiotic use in livestock. In the World Health Organization review of this intervention, a dramatic decrease in resistant bacteria was observed in animals, meat, and humans. In addition, eliminating the routine use of these antibiotics in livestock reduced human health risk without significantly harming the animals' health—and even the farmers' income did not suffer.

- For many years, hospitals would burn all of their waste in incinerators, and all of that material was being released into the atmosphere. Health Care Without Harm decided to take on this issue: In 1988, there were 6,200 medical waste incinerators in the United States, and by 2003, that number was down to 115.

- Health Care Without Harm is also behind the global ban of mercury. The Philippines, Argentina, Mexico, and other countries all over the globe are no longer using mercury—particularly mercury thermometers—because of their effort.

- In addition, Health Care Without Harm is working with hospitals to eliminate the use of PVC, which is a vinyl plastic that creates a number of environmental and health risks. Many health-care facilities around the world are switching to safer, more cost-effective medical devices that do not contain PVC.

- As a result of the Healthy Food in Health Care initiative, more than 350 hospitals have pledged to supply healthy, sustainable food to their patients and employees. Hospitals are making a commitment to use antibiotic-free meat and poultry and milk that is free of bovine growth hormone. Whenever possible, they are trying to offer foods that are certified organic. They are even trying to buy coffee that is fair trade, and they are filtering their water.

Questions to Consider

1. What is the difference between organic and nonorganic produce?

2. What potential toxin is found in plastic?

Healthy People, Healthy Planet
Lecture 23—Transcript

Welcome back. In the previous lecture, we discussed some key factors affecting the health of humans and the health of the planet. The news was pretty disheartening, and it served as a wakeup call to take action. Today's lecture is just about that, taking action.

Let's start with the concept to act locally. What can we do today, you and me, to impact not only our own health, but also the health of our planet?

Well, you have heard me say this before, one of the first things I want you to think about doing is to buy organic. Over 450 pesticides and herbicides are used on non-organic products. Non-organic products may be irradiated, they have nitrates, and the seeds may even be genetically modified, so whenever possible, buy organic. And there is another reason for this, if we keep using soil over and over and over again we deplete the soil of its nutrients. But organic farmers do what is called crop rotation, and it gives the soil more time to develop its nutrients again.

In the previous lecture, I reminded you about the Environmental Working Group. They have those fruits and vegetables that we really need to buy organic, remember we called it "The Dirty Dozen." Things like peaches, apples, sweet bell peppers, celery, nectarines, strawberries, cherries, pears, and grapes, and there are more. Those are the ones I really want you to focus on buying organic. Some of the thicker skinned products like onions and mangoes and pineapple, it kind of makes sense we can eat those non-organic. But also, quite frankly, we want to support our organic farmers; that is an added advantage.

A 2006 study revealed detectible metabolites of organophosphate pesticide residues in children eating a conventional diet. The really good news is that when these children were taken from the conventional diet and placed on an organic diet, there were no detectible metabolites. If the children were placed back on a conventional diet, the metabolites were detected again. So this is one quick solution, a choice that we can all make: to choose organic.

In addition to buying organic whenever possible, do your best to avoid eating meat and dairy. You have heard me say this over and over again; in the first place these foods are really high in saturated fat. We already said that the saturated fat contributes to heart disease, to inflammation. But, as we discussed in our last lecture, the industrialized reduction of livestock also leads to increased greenhouse gas admissions. So if we eat less meat and less dairy, it is actually improving our carbon footprint; we are polluting less, and that is a great thing. And we have lots of other good choices; we can have beans, lentils, and legumes as a great source of protein. This quick and easy substitution can be your individual contribution to decreasing greenhouse gas.

What else can we do? When you go to the supermarket, I want you to look for eggs that are free range and omega-3. That is what I want you to look for on the label. Why do I want them to be omega-3s? Because if an egg gets transported over a distance, the egg becomes pro-inflammatory, the omega-6 to omega-3 ratio is 15 or more to one. So we want to have the omega-3 back in the egg, and the egg you get on the farm is the freshest, best egg you can get. If you choose to eat poultry, I want you to look at the packaging here also, I want you to look for free-range, free of antibiotics and hormones, especially if you have small children. We do not want our children to be getting the hormones in the meat. So ideally, I would love for you to buy all of these products, the eggs, the poultry, organic.

As I have said in previous lectures, if choosing fish, make sure it is wild caught, such as wild sockeye salmon, the fatter a fish, the more fat on the fish, the more toxins in the fat, so choose a wild sockeye salmon or a wild trout, for example.

Speaking of fish, there is a clear difference between wild and farmed salmon, and a study came out in *Science* in 2004 where researchers found that farm-raised Atlantic salmon had significantly higher levels of 13 toxins when compared with wild Pacific salmon. What was interesting about this study is the same study also measured toxin levels in the salmon chow; this is what was fed to the salmon, a mixture of ground up fish and oil which was fed to the farm-raised salmon. They found a strong correlation between the toxicities of the chow and the salmon. Well this makes total sense. What they concluded was that the toxins are being passed into the salmon from their food.

So what I tell my patients is I say if you are going to eat an animal, even if it is salmon, I want you to ask a question of what did the animal eat? And I think you know by now that I want you to eat more legumes, beans, and lentils, and in general less animals.

An FDA veterinarian article gives some insight into what is going on in fish farms. They said that fish farms use chemicals as disinfectants to kill bacteria, they use herbicides to prevent the overgrowth of vegetation in the ponds, vaccines to fight certain diseases, and drugs, usually combined in the feed, to treat diseases and parasites. That is pretty scary stuff, and does not this remind us of what we talked about in a previous lecture, adding the antibiotics to the cow's food and the use of antibiotics in the agricultural industry?

Remember, when you make the decision to go and have fish, make sure it is wild and not farmed, and the sockeye, if you have salmon, is a good choice, because the sockeye eats algae.

We discussed some easy steps we can take, that promote not only our own health, but these steps promote the health of the planet as well. Let's take a look at a few more easy suggestions that can really make a big difference. And before I go there, you know that I want you to be vegan because that is the best food you can eat for the planet, and I bet a lot of you are saying "Oh, no, Dr. G., don't do it." Remember when we talked about BPA, which is in the plastic bottles? Well, I want you to start figuring out where in your bottles is there BPA, so flip your bottles over, look underneath, and if you see recycle number seven on the bottom, that bottle has BPA. But not everyone labels the bottles. So remember, most aluminum cans are lined with BPA, so whenever possible I want you to filter your water, remember that, and select stainless steel canisters, I want you not to put your hot foods in plastic, because if you put a hot food in a plastic container, the toxins from the plastic will go into the food, so stay away from hot foods and plastic, use glass, use porcelain, put your water in stainless steel containers, and one last thing: Do not microwave plastic, again for the same reason, when you microwave the plastic, the toxins from the plastic get into the food.

There is another issue with plastic; it's not just the BPA in the bottles. Those plastic bottles are ending up in the water, and of course, the environmental impact of plastic goes way beyond BPA. Let's take a look at this. We now know that plastic constitutes 90 percent of all trash floating in the world's oceans. Let me say that again, because this is kind of mind boggling, to me: Plastic constitutes 90 percent of all the trash floating in the world's oceans. The United Nations Environment program estimated in 2006 that every square mile of ocean hosts 46,000 pieces of floating plastic. In some areas of the ocean the amount of plastic outweighs the amount of plankton by a ratio of six to one.

I had never heard about the Pacific garbage patch until a couple of years ago, but there is actually something out there called the Pacific garbage patch. It is a trash vortex that spins around, it a gyre of ocean litter which is in the North Pacific Ocean. The exact size of the vortex is unknown, and estimates range from an area the size of the state of Texas to one larger than the continental United States. And there is one other sad piece to the plastic story, and this one really hurts me a lot to see: It is the albatross are dying because they are eating the plastic and they are eating the plastic bottle caps. So not only is it bad for us, not only is plastic bad for the planet, plastic is bad for the animals as well. So this is one that we really need to have a solution to immediately, and I am thrilled that people are giving up on their plastic bags, for example, I am really happy with that, I love when I see people going to the supermarket now and they have a cloth bag that they can reuse.

Did you know every year it takes 17 billion barrels of oil and produces 2.5 billion tons of carbon dioxide pollution to produce the 30 billion plastic bottles Americans use? That is crazy. It takes three times the amount of water to produce the bottle as it does to fill it. Now add to that the cost of transporting those heavy bottles, and this in no way adds up to environmental stewardship. So at the end of the day, we are going to filter our water.

I was at the airport a couple of weeks ago, and a guy went and bought a bottle of water. He was in front of me in the line, and he paid $5.12 for a bottle about yea big. And I said to him, "When did we reach a place in our life and in our society that we pay $5.12 for a bottle of water?" So please, when you go to work, filter your water at home, put it in that stainless steel bottle. This really helps us to avoid using the plastic; it prevents us from getting the exposure to the BPA, and if you absolutely must use plastic, recycle. But you know, a lot of people used to say to me, "Well I recycle my plastic," but look where it is ending up, it is ending up in the ocean. So obviously all that plastic is not getting recycled. So cut down its use as much as possible, because remember this: Plastic is forever.

I really hope I convinced you to put aside those plastic bottles, and I have to tell you one quick story. I gave a similar lecture as this to a group of Canadians, and about three months later, one of the men in the audience came to me and he said, "You know what I did?" I said, "What did you do?" He said, "I went to the head of my golf club, and I told them what you said about plastic. And so what the golf club has done is we all now have a stainless steel bottle with the name of the golf club on it and a guy just goes around with the cart and refills it with filtered water." One person changed the entire golf club. That is powerful medicine. One person could do that; imagine if all of us did these contributions? And I have one last recommendation; I want you to walk instead of drive. Sounds so simple, walking is medicine and improves everything from our weight to our cholesterol to our depression, remember we said exercise helps us sleep better? So if we choose to walk or bike instead of driving, not only do we help ourselves, but that is a perfect way to help the planet.

So far we have been discussing those things that we can do as individuals. I am going to say it again: We could all be vegan. I want to get rid of the dairy, if you can, and especially that red meat. We can filter our water, we do not have to buy plastic bottles, and we certainly do not have to drink from them. Now let's look at some other changes that are happening at a little larger level, both institutionally and nationally.

In our last lecture we talked about misuse of antibiotics in livestock. You are probably tired of me saying this. We should not give animals that do not have infection antibiotics. It leads to antibiotic-resistant bacteria. Well, one country has taken steps to solve this problem, and that is Denmark. In

1998 Denmark eliminated non-therapeutic antibiotic use in livestock. In the World Health Organization review of this intervention, a dramatic decrease in resistant bacteria was observed in animals, meat, and humans. What more do we need? A decrease in resistant bacteria in animals, meat, and humans. This is exactly what we want to see, just by eliminating the non-therapeutic use of antibiotics. In addition, eliminating the routine use of these antibiotics in livestock reduced human health risk without significantly harming the animals' health. Even the farmers' income did not suffer.

Denmark is a great example of what can happen if we change policy. And policy change is a big piece of this puzzle. But as we have seen, individuals can affect change very quickly, like getting rid of the plastic bags. So we need to tackle this problem from a couple of different directions. As a physician I am really pleased to say that medical professionals as a group are taking some really good positive steps toward improving the health of the planet.

One organization that is having an incredible impact is Health Care Without Harm. You may not think a lot about this, but for years, hospitals would pile all of their waste, IV bags, pumps, anything that they could in incinerators and burn the material. All of that material was being released into the atmosphere. Health Care Without Harm decided to take on this issue. In 1988 there were 6200 medical waste incinerators in the United States. By 2003 that number was down to 115. That is the power of what a group coming together can do. Health Care Without Harm has also done some other interesting things; they have been singlehandedly behind the global ban of mercury particularly in health-care systems. The Philippines, Argentina, Mexico, countries all over the globe are no longer using mercury, particularly mercury thermometers, because of their effort. And a third success that they are working on right now, they are working with hospitals to eliminate the use of PVC, that is vinyl plastic, and it is used everywhere in health-care. Think about this: IV bags are plastic, disposable gloves, curtains, even hospital flooring is made of PVC. The use of PVC creates a number of environmental and health risks, due to these concerns many health-care facilities around the world are switching now to safer, cost-effective medical devices that do not have vinyl plastic, and bravo to Health Care Without Harm for leading the way.

The partnership between hospitals and Health Care Without Harm is really making a difference. And another positive development is the Healthy Food in health-care initiative. I remember when I was stenting in the '90s and I would put the stent in and my patients would go up to their room in the hospital and they would get a roast beef and mayo sandwich on white bread. Three great food groups for someone with heart disease. But today, more than 350 hospitals have pledged to supply healthy and sustainable food to their patients and employees. Hospitals are making a commitment to use antibiotic-free meat and poultry. They are making a commitment to use milk that is free of bovine growth hormone. Whenever possible, they are trying to give foods that are certified organic. They are even trying to get coffee, for example, that is fair trade. This is incredible, and they are filtering their water. I was thrilled when Scripps decided to put in a water filtering system. Not only is the water better, but we no longer have those big plastic bottles sitting around anymore.

There are many hospitals I can talk about here, but I just picked one, because it illustrates what a little bit of policy change can do, and that is the Dominican Hospital in Santa Cruz. Since 2005 patient menus have been completely redesigned. They are intentionally making more healthy recipes. Let me tell you what one of their recipes is: Thai basil tofu and spinach. If that's whole foods/organic, that's a perfect food; roasted garlic and tomato soup; they have quinoa, a wonderful grain, on the menu. This to me is going to transform everything. I always wondered why we served bad food in hospitals, and I remember once my aunt said to me, "I got eggs when I was in the hospital, so I assumed they were good for me." So what people get in the hospital, they do think is good for them, and this is setting a new, wonderful message. The menus at Dominican are frequently vegetarian or vegan; there is always an option. There is one other fun thing happening at the Dominican Hospital in Santa Cruz, the hospital chef cooks with produce from the hospital's garden. That is great, that is perfect. Their produce does not have to travel anywhere; it goes from the earth to the plate. So local produce means less pollution, and those things that he is not growing he is sourcing from the surrounding farms. And this has the added benefit of supporting the local community. Dominican also has a very large compost program, so they are recycling in environmentally friendly way.

I have to share one hospital that is not in the United States, so we have our United States sample. This is the Changi General Hospital in Singapore. This to me was really insightful. This hospital grows hydroponic plants on the rooftop, which provide food for the hospital. But what also happens is these plants help to absorb the heat making naturally ventilated wards much cooler. That is incredibly insightful. They grow lots of different fruits and vegetables but one year they produced 190 kg of cherry tomatoes.

This is a concept that is really beginning to take hold: It is called green roofing. I like to think about it this way: If we take something from the earth, if we take a piece of the earth, especially if we are going to build on it, we have to put it up on the roof, and that is what we are seeing happening in many places around the world.

So clearly, the health-care community is doing something that you can tell I am excited about. Hospitals are finally making a shift from being illness-focused to actually places of health. Remember we said in the beginning that the key is to get to the underlying cause of medical problems? These choices are getting to the underlying cause, because they are choices that are healthy for people and also healthy for the planet.

Today we have seen that human health is connected to the health of the planet in a very meaningful and special way. When we make those right choices for our own health, we are also making choices that are right for planet Earth. Truly what is personal is universal.

You Are Your Own Best Medicine
Lecture 24

Throughout this course, you have learned about a new paradigm of health that supports the notion that prevention is the best intervention. The new paradigm treats the whole person—body, mind, emotions, and spirit—reaches the underlying cause of disease, and strengthens the soil in which a person lives. You have learned how the science of natural healing gives you powerful tools to achieve optimal health. In this lecture, you will learn that the secret ingredient is actually you—because you are your own best medicine.

What Makes People Heal?
- Jerome Frank was a physician, psychotherapy researcher, folk healer, and even an antinuclear activist. In 1961, he wrote a book called *Persuasion and Healing*. Dr. Frank's work sought to answer the question: What makes people heal? The following conclusions resulted from his work.

- Dr. Frank believed that healing requires the patient and physician to share the belief that healing will occur. Healing also requires an emotionally charged setting, a confiding relationship, and some kind of ritual surrounding the healing event. In addition, Dr. Frank said that healing requires hope.

- The word "placebo" is used to describe any form of treatment in which patients are led to believe that they are experiencing a beneficial procedure or receiving a curative agent when, in reality, they are being given something that has no known healing properties.

- A study was published in the *Journal of Affective Disorders* to evaluate the impact of the psychotherapist on treating patients with depression. Their objective was not to evaluate the depression treatment as much as the psychotherapist. People were placed into two groups: One group received a placebo, and the second group received an active drug. The difference was the therapist. Those people who had a caring, empathetic therapist—even though they received the placebo—did better than the individuals who had a less caring therapist and received an active drug.

- A similar study was conducted to evaluate the impact of a physician's empathy on the ability to control patients' diabetes and cholesterol. Physicians were ranked as having high, moderate, or low empathy. Those physicians who were ranked as having the highest empathy had the most success controlling their patients' diabetes and cholesterol.

- Dr. Irving Kirsch, Director of the Program in Placebo Studies at Harvard Medical School, believes that all responses are based on expectancy. In essence, what we expect will indeed occur.

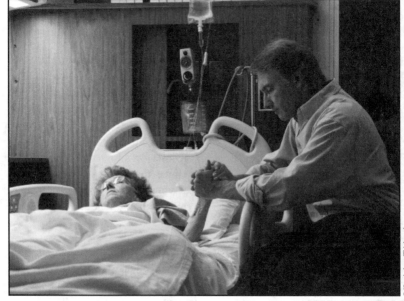

There is great power in believing that you will heal—and in others believing that you will heal.

- In 2002, a study was published in which 17 men with major depression were randomized to receive either an active placebo or the antidepression medication Prozac. PET scans of the brain were performed to look at brain activity and to evaluate different brain patterns associated with different emotions and psychiatric illnesses. The patients were scanned before and after the study. Similar brain changes were seen in the placebo and medication group.

- These studies demonstrate the power of ritual and expectation to bring about healing.

- Sometimes, patients express unfounded beliefs to their physicians that they will develop an illness or die as a result of a medication or treatment. These beliefs lead to what is known as a nocebo reaction or response, which refers to the harmful, unpleasant, or undesirable effects that occur after a patient receives a medication or treatment. A nocebo response is caused by the subject's pessimistic beliefs and expectations that the placebo will produce negative consequences.

- The Framingham Heart Study—directed by the National Heart, Lung, and Blood Institute and Boston University—enrolled 5,290 men and women from Framingham, Massachusetts, between the ages of 30 and 62. The purpose of this research was to follow these patients over a long period of time in order to identify factors associated with coronary artery disease. The researchers were surprised to find that women who believed they were prone to heart disease at the start of the study were almost four times more likely to die as those with similar risk factors who did not hold this belief.

- Belief is not simply thought; it goes much deeper than that, and it is much more complex. Belief can best be defined as the certainty that comes from accepting what we think is true in our minds as well as what we feel to be true in our hearts. Belief is at the very core of our being.

- The women in the Framingham Heart Study were convinced that they would get heart disease, and they focused on what they believed to be true—that they would get heart disease. Could it be that they actually manifested this reality? Is it possible that we create the things in life that mirror our own thoughts and feelings? More importantly, what happens if we change that thinking and bring in a new perspective?

- Affirmations provide a way to change your thinking. An affirmation is a declaration that something is true. It is not about just saying words; it is about knowing with your mind and believing in your heart that what you are saying is true. For example, the declaration "I am healed" is a positive affirmation. It is not a declaration in the past tense or in the future tense; instead, the healing is happening in the present moment.

- In 2007, David Creswell conducted a study to evaluate the effect of affirmations through expressive writing in breast cancer survivors. When the essays written by the women were analyzed, the author concluded that women whose writings were affirmative experienced fewer negative symptoms and a better health outcome.

What Have You Learned?
- Throughout this course, you have explored the big picture that connects the health of the planet to the choices that you make every day as an individual.

- You have uncovered the importance of tiny molecules such as vitamin D to your body and mind.

- You have learned about nutrition, exercise, meditation, and service.

- You have examined the evidence that supports the health benefits of love, forgiveness, and connection.

- You have observed the power of thought. Thoughts truly can make us sick, but they can also make us well.

- There are many paths to healing, and the path may be different for each person.

- You have the power to be your own best medicine.

- Hopefully, this course has provided you with all of the necessary tools, science, and wisdom to start your healing journey. Information leads to knowledge, but practice leads to transformation.

Questions to Consider

1. What is a placebo?

2. How are belief and expectation linked to health?

You Are Your Own Best Medicine
Lecture 24—Transcript

In 1939 a surgical procedure was performed to treat coronary artery disease. The procedure was called mammary artery ligation. Basically, what the surgeons did was cut the artery that runs down the chest wall. This procedure was thought to improve blood flow to the heart, and was performed for 20 years as a routine treatment for heart disease.

Twenty years later, the surgery was compared to a sham operation. Patients received a surgical cut on their chest, but the artery was never actually touched. The medical community was shocked when the patients receiving the sham procedure had the same success rates as those who actually had the intervention. The surgeons had to accept the fact that the surgery they had been performing for the last 20 years was no better than a placebo.

The word placebo is used to describe any form of treatment where patients are led to believe that they are experiencing a beneficial procedure or receiving a curative agent while in reality they are giving something that has no known healing properties.

A more recent study of sham surgery was conducted by a group of orthopedic surgeons. The condition under study was knee pain. Patients were placed in three different groups, two of the groups received an actual surgical intervention, and the third group received a sham procedure. Again, the results showed that people in the placebo group did as well as the people in the treatment group. The knee pain in all three groups improved equally.

In both of these sham surgery studies it is important to note that patients were truly led to believe that they were undergoing surgery. Patients were placed under surgical anesthesia, an actual incision was made, and they recovered in the hospital. Needless to say, these kinds of experiments are not being done today.

The charged elements of going to the hospital and having a procedure increased the placebo response because the participant believes they are getting a real surgery. But, the sham surgery is basically a fake operation. All the steps are identical to the real procedure with the exception of the actual therapeutic intervention.

While one group received surgery and one did not, both groups of people believed they received treatment. They believed they received treatment, and it was revealed that the key is belief.

Over the past 23 lectures we have seen how the science of natural healing gives us powerful tools to achieve optimal health. Now it appears that the secret ingredient is actually you. At the end of the day, you are your own best medicine.

Jerome Frank was a physician; he was also a psychotherapy researcher, a folk healer, and even an anti-nuclear activist. He wrote a book in 1961 called *Persuasion and Healing*. Dr. Frank's work sought to answer the question of what makes people heal. From his work come the following conclusions.

Dr. Frank believed that healing required the patient and physician to share the belief that healing would occur. Healing also requires an emotionally charged setting and a confiding relationship. But Dr. Frank did not stop there. He went on to say that healing also requires some kind of ritual surrounding the healing event. Remember the ritual surrounding the sham surgery? The patients really believed they were having an operation. In this case the surgery was the ritual. In addition, Dr. Frank said that healing requires hope.

When I think of Dr. Frank's principles of what makes people heal, I am reminded of my own medical practice. I can't help but to think of my patient Herb. Herb was a senior corporate executive who had lots of medical problems. Herb had really severe heart disease. Herb came to see me on his 85th birthday, and asked me if I would write a clearance for him to go and have surgery. When I asked Herb why he needed to have surgery, he lifted his right hand to show me that he had damage to a tendon. Herb was unable to lift his third digit, so it became very hard for him to write. I really did not want to send Herb to surgery, he had so many medical problems, and I was concerned about the anesthesia. I was afraid that Herb's surgery might result in a complication.

I asked Herb if he would like for me to do a Healing Touch treatment, and he said yes. For 20 minutes he and I remained quiet as I performed Healing Touch on his upper extremity. Herb left the appointment with a smile. I gave him a big hug, and I also gave him his surgical clearance. Three days later I was really surprised to receive a call from Herb. He said, "Guess what, Dr. G.? My surgery was cancelled. You cured me."

Now, I do not believe for one minute that I cured Herb. Like the surgical procedure, seeing a physician in the office can also be a very emotionally charged situation. I learned a long time ago that even the handing of a prescription to a patient will have an effect on their response to that medication. Let me give you an example: When I was a younger physician, I would give a patient a medication and I would say, "Why don't we try this medication? Let's see how you do." Even though I knew intellectually that this was the best medication at the time for the problem. I subsequently realized that if I believed that something really was going to work I needed to put my energy into that prescription and hand it to the patient in a different way. So now when I hand a patient a prescription, I say, "This is going to work." What bigger ritual do we have that happens thousands of times a day in hospitals and physicians offices all over the world, the act of handing a patient a prescription and telling them that it will make them well sets in motion the patient's own intent to heal.

With Herb, the Healing Touch treatment was the ritual. And I will never know what healed Herb's hand, whether his healing was from Healing Touch, placebo, or the hug that I gave him at the end of the appointment. I do not really need to know. All I know is he never had a problem with that hand again.

Herb was not a patient that I had seen for the first time. Herb and I had a very special relationship. Herb had been my patient for many years. We had a lot of history together. There is no doubt that we had bonded. I loved him as a human being, and I know that he knew that. I was really torn that day because I didn't want him to have to go and have a surgery; I didn't want him to potentially have a complication. The Healing Touch treatment was as much for him as it was for me, because I felt like I needed to do something

for Herb. To me, that is the nature of the patent-phys¹
that does not always go on in a medical office.

What happens if a physician is not empathetic'
of close, confiding relationship? A study was publi.
Affective Disorders to evaluate the impact of the psychotn.
patients with depression. Their objective was not to evaluate u.
treatment as much as the psychotherapist. People were placed ш.
groups: One group received a placebo and the second an active drug. т.
difference was the therapist. What they found was of course amazing. Those
people, who had a caring, empathetic therapist, even though they got the
placebo, did better than the individuals who had a less-caring therapist, even
though those individuals received an active drug.

A similar study was conducted to evaluate the impact of a physician's
empathy on the ability to control patients' diabetes and cholesterol.
Physicians were ranked as having high, moderate, or low empathy. No
surprises, those physicians ranked as having the highest empathy had the
most success controlling their patients' diabetes and cholesterol. What I have
seen in my practice is my patients frequently come in and say to me, "Dr. G.,
I lost 10 pounds for you," and I laugh to myself because it makes me happy,
and of course I am glad they improved their weight, but it is for them as well.
But the fact that they would do it for me really touches my heart.

Irving Kirsch, Director of the Program in Placebo Studies at Harvard Medical
School believes that all responses are based on expectancy. In essence, what
we expect will indeed occur.

Let's look at one more fascinating study. In 2002, a study was published in
which 17 men with major depression were randomized to receive an active
placebo or the antidepression medication Prozac. PET scans of the brain
were performed to look at brain activity. The PET scans were to evaluate
different brain patterns associated with different emotions and psychiatric
illnesses. The patients were scanned before and after the study. Similar brain
changes were seen in the placebo and medication group. PET scans where
areas of the brain lit up were the same. The authors concluded, and I quote,

efore emphasized that administration of placebo is not absence of
ht, just an absence of active medication."

have seen the power of ritual and expectation to bring about healing. That
what these studies are telling us. But what happens if a patient believes
hat they will develop an illness, or if a patient believes that they will die?
This is referred to as "nocebo."

In medicine, a nocebo reaction or response refers to harmful, unpleasant, or undesirable effects after receiving a medication or treatment. A nocebo response is due to the subject's pessimistic beliefs and expectation that the placebo will produce negative consequences.

I remember once when I was a young physician, I offered a patient a medication for his diabetes, and he quickly told me that he did not want to take that medication, and I quote, "Doc, I do not want to take that medicine. It is going to kill me." He did not really know anything about the drug, he had never even heard about this medicine. So I insisted he take the medication. I told him it was one of the best medicines on the market. Well, he took the medication, and had a profound allergic reaction. Fortunately for my patient he was fine in the end, but this taught me, as a physician, a really good lesson. Again, I am not certain whether he actually had an allergic reaction to the drug, or whether he manifested the allergic reaction by truly believing that he was going to die. Or maybe he even had an inner knowing, what I call your own inner physician that clued in him on his own vulnerability. Either way, I now have the greatest respect for my patients' intuition.

Is there any research to validate the concept that what we believe can have negative consequences? Let's take a look. The Framingham Heart Study directed by the National Heart Institute enrolled 5290 men and women from Framingham, Massachusetts, between the ages of 30 and 62. Thousands of papers have been published from the Framingham Heart Study. The purpose of this research was to follow these patients over a long period of time, to identify factors associated with coronary artery disease. The researchers were surprised to find that women who believed they were prone to heart disease at the start of the study were almost four times more likely to die as those with similar risk factors who did not hold this belief.

In the case of the Framingham Heart Study, these women believed they were going to get sick. Belief is not simply thought, it goes much deeper than that, and it is much more complex.

Belief can best be defined as the certainty that comes from accepting what we think is true in our minds as well as what we feel to be true in our hearts. Belief is at the very core of our being.

The women in the Framingham Heart Study were convinced that they would get heart disease. These women focused on what they believed to be true, that they would get heart disease. Could it be that they actually manifested this reality? Is it possible that we create the things in life that mirror our own thoughts and feelings? And, more importantly, what happens if we change that thinking? What happens when we bring in a new perspective?

Affirmations are a way of doing just that. An affirmation is a declaration that something is true, it is not about just saying words, it is about knowing with your mind and believing in your heart what you are saying. Let me give you an example: "I am healed," is a positive affirmation. It is not the past tense, or the future tense, it is not "I am going to be healed," it is "I am healed, I am whole." The healing happens right there in the present moment. So we have seen that stress can make us sick, but now we know that what we believe can also make us well.

David Creswell in 2007 conducted a study to evaluate the effect of affirmations through expressive writing in breast cancer survivors. When the essays written by the women were analyzed, the author concluded that women whose writings were affirmative, experienced fewer negative symptoms, and a better health outcome.

When I think of the power of affirmations, I have to tell one more story about my patient, Harry. I have been Harry's physician for at least 15 years. He came to see me about 15 years ago and was having some shortness of breath. I did a full evaluation, even a coronary angiogram. I told Harry that I thought it would be best if he had a bypass. Harry said to me, "Bypass?" I said, "Yes, open heart surgery." And he looked at me and he said, "Dr. G., I am not having a bypass. I have things to do." And this is exactly what he said. He said, "I have six bunny rabbits at home that I have to feed, and every Friday, I have to meet my friends to fly my model planes. I am not having a bypass." And then Harry said, "Dr. G., I do not need a bypass." I stepped back a bit, and I thought eventually, I will talk Harry into this bypass surgery.

So I took his angiogram to what we call Cardiology Conference, and I had the entire angiogram reviewed with my colleagues. And 20 out of 20 cardiologists in the room said Harry needed a bypass. So when Harry came back to see me, I said, "Harry, the entire committee, every cardiologist we have says you need a bypass. And I agree." And he looked at me again, and said, "Dr. G., I do not need a bypass." But he came from a really deep place. This was not just saying words; he meant it. Well, you know how this story ends, because it is 15 years later and Harry still hasn't had his bypass.

Through the science of natural healing, we have discussed a new paradigm of health. We have concluded that prevention is the best intervention. The new paradigm treats the whole person, body, mind, emotions, and spirit. The new paradigm gets to the underlying cause of disease, and strengthens the soil in which we live.

We have explored the big picture that connects the health of the planet to the choices that we make every day as individuals. And, we have zoomed in on tiny molecules like vitamin D, revealing their importance to our bodies and to our mind. We have talked about nutrition, exercise, meditation, and service. We have examined the evidence that supports the health benefits of love, of forgiveness, and the health benefits of connection, and we concluded that the W E in wellness is we. And today, once again, we have seen the power of thought. Thoughts, we discovered, really can make us sick. But, if they can make us sick, our thoughts can also make us well. There are many paths to healing and the path may be different for each of us. But, whatever path you take, remember this: You have the power to be your own best medicine. It is my personal hope that the science of natural healing provides you with all the necessary tools, science, and wisdom to start your healing journey. Remember, information leads to knowledge, but practice will lead to transformation.

Bibliography

Integrative Medicine Resources
Guarneri, M. *The Heart Speaks: A Cardiologist Reveals the Secret Language of Healing.* New York: Touchstone, 2006.

Rakel, David. *Integrative Medicine.* Philadelphia: Saunders, 2002.

Spiegel, Bernie S. *Love, Medicine, and Miracles: Lessons Learned about Self-Healing from a Surgeon's Experience with Exceptional Patients.* New York: William Morrow Paperback, 1990.

Stress Resources
Childre, Doc, and Deborah Rozman. *Transforming Stress: The Heartmath Solution for Relieving Worry, Fatigue, and Tension.* Oakland, CA: New Harbinger Publications, 2005.

Easwaran, Eknath. *Strength in the Storm: Creating Calm in Difficult Times.* Tomales, CA: Nilgiri Press, 2005.

Kabat-Zinn, Jon. *Wherever You Go, There You Are: Mindfulness Meditation in Everyday Life.* 10th anniversary ed. New York: Hyperion, 2005.

Pearsall, Paul. *Toxic Success: How to Stop Striving and Start Thriving.* Makawao, HI: Inner Ocean Publishing, 2002.

Selye, Hans. *The Stress of Life.* 2nd ed. Columbus, OH: McGraw-Hill, 1978.

Nutrition Resource
Pratt, Steven G., and Kathy Matthews. *SuperFoods Rx: Fourteen Foods That Will Change Your Life.* New York: William Morrow Paperback, 2005.

Heart Disease Resource
Ornish, Dean. *Dr. Dean Ornish's Program for Reversing Heart Disease.* New York: Ballantine Books, 1992.

Spirituality Resources

Ellerby, Jonathan H. *Return to the Sacred: Ancient Pathways to Spiritual Awakening*. New York: Hay House, 2010.

Muller, Wayne. *How, Then, Shall We Live?: Four Simple Questions That Reveal the Beauty and Meaning of Our Lives*. New York, Bantam, 1997.

Tolle, Eckhart. *The Power of Now: A Guide to Spiritual Enlightenment*. Novato, CA: New World Library, 2004.

Mind-Body Resource

Moyers, Bill. *Healing and the Mind*. St. Charles, MO: Main Street Books, 1995.

Environmental Resource

Gaynor, Mitchell. *Nurture Nature, Nurture Health: Your Health and the Environment*. New York: Nurture Nature Press, 2005.

Internet Resources

American Board of Integrative Holistic Medicine. Accessed May 1, 2012. www.abihm.org.

American Botanical Council. Accessed May 1, 2012. www.herbalgram.org.

The Bravewell Collaborative. Accessed May 1, 2012. www.bravewell.org.

ConsumerLab.com. Accessed May 1, 2012. www.consumerlab.com.

Environmental Working Group. Accessed May 1, 2012. www.ewg.org.

The Institute for Functional Medicine. Accessed May 1, 2012. www.functionalmedicine.org.

Mimi Guarneri, M.D., FACC. Accessed May 1, 2012. www.mimiguarnerimd.com.

National Center for Complementary and Alternative Medicine. Accessed May 1, 2012. nccam.nih.gov.

National Institutes of Health, Office of Dietary Supplements. Accessed May 1, 2012. ods.od.nih.gov.

Natural Medicines Comprehensive Database. Accessed May 1, 2012. www.naturaldatabase.com.

Scripps Center for Integrative Medicine, Scripps Health. Accessed May 1, 2012. www.scrippsintegrativemedicine.org.

U.S. Department of Health & Human Services, U.S. Food and Drug Administration. MedWatch: The FDA Safety Information and Adverse Event Reporting Program. Accessed May 1, 2012. www.fda.gov/medwatch.

Notes

Notes

Notes

Notes

Notes

Notes

Notes